Preface

Incontinence is one of the four 'giants of geriatric medicine', the others being intellectual impairment, instability and immobility. It is the 'giant' with which most physicians are least familiar. This is because much of the published work is to be found in surgical or nursing journals and textbooks. This book is written from the perspective of a physician specializing in the care of the elderly. Although most of the book is concerned with urinary incontinence the final two chapters are devoted to the less common, but equally important problem, of faecal incontinence. I would like to thank Dr James Barratt for his help and advice in the preparation of these chapters.

Gerald W Tobin
Bristol, January 1992

Incontinence in the elderly

Gerald W. Tobin

MD, FRCPI

Consultant Physician, Care of the Elderly,
The United Bristol Healthcare NHS Trust

Edward Arnold

A division of Hodder & Stoughton
LONDON MELBOURNE AUCKLAND

© 1992 Gerald W. Tobin

First published in Great Britain 1992

British Library Cataloguing in Publication Data
Tobin, Gerald W.
  Incontinence in the Elderly
  I. Title
  618.97

  ISBN 0–340–54558–5

Whilst the advice and information in this book is believed to be true and accurate at the date of going to press, neither the author nor the publisher can accept any legal responsibility or liability for any errors or omissions that may be made. In particular (but without limiting the generality of the preceding disclaimer) every effort has been made to check drug dosages; however, it is still possible that errors have been missed. Furthermore, dosage schedules are constantly being revised and new side effects recognised. For these reasons the reader is strongly urged to consult the drug companies' printed instructions before administering any of the drugs recommended in this book.

Typeset in 10 on 12 pt Times by Wearset, Boldon, Tyne and Wear. Printed in Great Britain for Edward Arnold, a division of Hodder and Stoughton Limited, Mill Road, Dunton Green, Sevenoaks, Kent TN13 2YA by St Edmundsbury Press Ltd, Bury St Edmunds, Suffolk, and bound by Hartnolls Ltd, Bodmin, Cornwall.

Contents

1 The anatomy and physiology of the lower urinary
   tract   1
2 The pathophysiology of urinary incontinence   10
3 Epidemiological and psychological aspects of
   incontinence   25
4 Diagnosis and the use of urodynamic
   investigations   29
5 Voiding regimes   46
6 The drug treatment of urinary incontinence   52
7 Surgical treatment of incontinence   62
8 Other aspects of management   70
9 Physiology of defecation   80
10 Faecal incontinence   88
Index   92

Chapter 1 _____

The anatomy and physiology of the lower urinary tract

The bladder and urethra can be considered as one unit with two parts, each of which has two functions. The bladder stores and then expels urine. It retains large volumes of urine but at low pressure, allowing urine to continue to enter from the ureters and keeping the pressure in the bladder lower than that in the urethra during the storage phase. The bladder expels its contents, at a convenient time and in an appropriate location, leaving no residual urine. The urethra offers resistance and then conveys. Continence requires that the pressure in the urethra exceed that in the bladder except during voluntary micturition. The urethra must maintain a pressure greater than that in the bladder not only at rest but also under conditions of stress. It lowers its resistance just before and during voluntary micturition.

The bladder

The empty bladder lies behind the pubic symphysis and is largely a pelvic organ (Fig. 1). The wall of the bladder has an outer coat of connective tissue, a smooth muscle layer and an inner mucous membrane. The muscle coat, referred to as the detrusor muscle, consists of interlacing bundles of smooth muscle cells. Although there are no discrete layers of muscle cells, longitudinally orientated bundles tend to predominate on the outer and inner aspects. The base of the bladder is thicker than the rest and thus undergoes less distension during filling. Contraction of the detrusor causes a reduction in all dimensions of the bladder lumen.

The trigone is a triangular area bounded superiorly by the ureteric orifices and inferiorly by the internal urethral orifice. The ureteric orifices are joined by the inter-ureteric ridge. The smooth muscle of the trigone consists of two layers, the superficial and deep trigone. The smooth muscle of the deep trigone is a continuation of the detrusor muscle. The superficial trigone is a thin, morphologically distinct, muscle layer. Its muscle cells are of smaller diameter than those of the remainder of the detrusor and are continuous

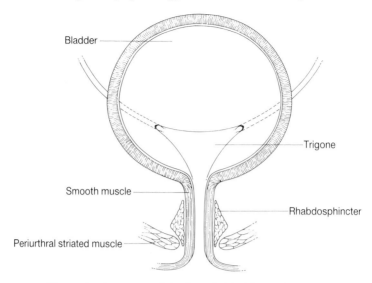

Figure 1   Anatomy of the female bladder and urethra.

proximally with those of the intramural ureters and distally with those of the urethra. In the male the smooth muscle cells of the bladder neck form a circular collar which extends distally to the pre-prostatic urethra. In contrast, in the female the muscle bundles extend obliquely or longitudinally into the proximal urethra. The mucosa of the bladder consists of a lining of transitional epithelium over a layer of connective tissue.

The urethra

The mucosa of the urethra is lined by transitional, pseudostratified columnar or stratified squamous epithelium depending on the level. In the female the squamous epithelium moves proximally with increasing age. The mucosa of the urethra is arranged in longitudinal folds.

When the urethra is closed its lumen has a stellate appearance in cross-section. This arrangement allows for considerable urethral dilatation. The muscle coat consists of smooth and striated muscle. The smooth muscle is arranged as an inner longitudinal layer surrounded by a thin circular layer. The striated muscle surrounds the smooth muscle layer and is called the rhabdosphincter. It is thickest in the anterior wall and at the mid-urethra in the female. It is anatomically distinct from the adjacent striated muscle of the pelvic floor from which it is separated by a layer of connective tissue. Its fibres are capable of sustained contraction. The periurethral striated muscle of the pelvic floor can contract quickly, as on coughing or on voluntary interruption of the urinary stream, but cannot maintain a sustained contraction. The male urethra is divided into the pre-prostatic urethra, the prostatic urethra, the membranous urethra and the spongiose urethra.

Peripheral innervation of the lower urinary tract

Efferent parasympathetic nerve supply

The preganglionic fibres arise in the intermediolateral region of the second to fourth segments of the sacral cord. The fibres travel via the pelvic nerves, joining the hypogastric nerves to form the vesical plexus. The vesical plexus is an extension of the pelvic plexus on to the lateral surface of the bladder. The preganglionic fibres synapse with the postganglionic fibres near the bladder wall. Within the bladder, nerves pursue a tortuous course, enabling them to accommodate to being stretched during bladder filling. The neural transmitter released by both the preganglionic and postganglionic neurones is acetylcholine. These cholinergic nerves are evenly distributed to all parts of the bladder except for the superficial trigone which has a sparse supply. They are responsible for detrusor contraction. They supply the entire length of the urethra in the female. In the male they innervate the urethra as far as the entrance of the ejaculatory ducts.

Efferent sympathetic nerve supply

The efferent sympathetic nerve supply arises in the interomediolateral grey columns of the thoracolumbar spinal cord from the tenth thoracic to the second lumbar segment. The preganglionic neurones pass to the inferior mesenteric plexus. From there they pass to the hypogastric plexus and join the pelvic nerves forming the vesical plexus. The neurotransmitter released by the preganglionic neurones is acetylcholine, whereas that released by the postganglionic neurones is noradrenaline.

The superficial trigonal muscle has a plentiful sympathetic supply. The adrenoceptors of the superficial trigone are mainly α-adrenoceptors. The remainder of the detrusor has a sparse sympathetic innervation. These are mainly β-adrenoceptors mediating relaxation. In the male the proximal urethra and bladder neck have a rich sympathetic innervation. These are mainly α-adrenoceptors mediating smooth muscle contraction. It has been postulated that their function is to prevent reflux ejaculation. In contrast few noradrenergic neurones have been identified in the proximal urethra of the female. This was an unexpected finding as pharmacological studies indicate α-adrenoceptor sites in this region in the female. The explanation for this may be that postganglionic sympathetic nerves synapse on postganglionic parasympathetic nerves where they have an inhibitory effect. Thus sympathetic effects may be mediated via an effect on parasympathetic ganglionic transmission.

The peripheral innervation of the rhabdosphincter is controversial. It is generally considered to be innervated by somatic fibres which travel via the pudendal nerve. Some authors believe that the rhabdosphincter also has an α-adrenergic supply.

The importance of the sympathetic nerve supply for the normal functioning of the lower urinary tract is unclear. Agents which stimulate or block α-adrenoceptors on the human urethra can produce significant changes in intraurethral pressure. It is also known that the relaxing effect obtained by stimulating the β-adrenoceptors on the bladder wall is small. Most authorities consider the sympathetic nervous system to have a very minor role in the functioning of the lower urinary tract. Those who consider it to have an important role believe its main function is to facilitate the storage phase of the micturition cycle by increasing outlet resistance and inhibiting bladder contractility.

The branches of the efferent autonomic nerves to the bladder have swellings called varicosities. Vesicles within a varicosity contain neurotransmitters. Three types of vesicle can be identified by electron microscopy. Vesicles containing acetylcholine are agranular. Noradrenaline is held in small dense cored vesicles. Large dense cored vesicles can also be identified. The neurotransmitter they contain is unknown. It may be a neural peptide, perhaps vasoactive intestinal polypeptide, and may be responsible for modifying the contractility of the detrusor smooth muscle.

Efferent somatic supply

The periurethral striated muscles of the pelvic floor are supplied by somatic fibres which originate in the anterior horn cells of the second to fourth sacral segments and travel via the pudendal nerve. The innervation of the rhabdosphincter has already been discussed.

Afferent nerves

These travel with the parasympathetic, sympathetic and somatic nerves. Afferents from the muscle coat are thought to travel mainly to the sacral region of the cord while afferents arising in the submucosa travel mainly to the lumbar region. Afferents from the muscle coat respond to an increase in bladder wall tension, resulting either from bladder distension or contraction. Individual detrusor receptors climb to a maximum firing rate which then remains constant. The individual receptors have different thresholds. Thus by recruiting different receptors at different levels of pressure the afferent system can indicate the pressure status of the bladder. In the spinal cord these proprioceptive fibres travel in the posterior column. Afferents arising in the mucosa convey touch, pain and temperature sensation. They are thought to travel in the spinothalamic tracts.

Neural control of lower urinary tract function

Although afferents from the bladder synapse on interneurones involved in a variety of spinal reflexes it is now known that the critical neural circuit involved in the control of micturition relays through the brain stem (Fig. 2).

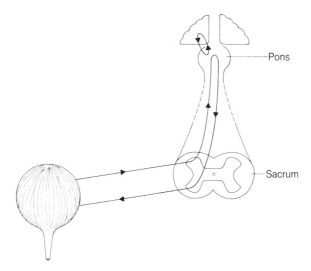

Figure 2 Neurological control of the lower urinary tract.

This is referred to as the long routing detrusor reflex. Sensory afferents from the detrusor synapse on projection neurones in the spinal cord. These neurones ascend to the brainstem detrusor nucleus believed to be located in the nucleus locus coeruleus in the pons. Efferent pathways arising in this area travel to the intermediolateral regions of the tenth thoracic to second lumbar segments and the second to fourth sacral segments of the spinal cord. The principle descending pathway is in the lateral reticulospinal tract and produces excitation in the preganglionic parasympathetic neurones along with inhibition of the neurones supplying the smooth and striated muscles of the urethra. A second pathway descends in the medial reticulospinal tract and inhibits the neurones of the striated external sphincter. A third pathway which descends in the ventral reticulospinal tract inhibits the preganglionic parasympathetic neurones as well as exciting the neurones to the urethra.

This long routed detrusor reflex ensures coordination between the action of the detrusor and the urethra. Detrusor contraction is accompanied by relaxation of the smooth and striated muscles of the urethra. Interruption of this reflex leads to detrusor sphincter dyssynergia. This term describes a detrusor contraction which is accompanied by an inappropriate contraction of the urethral and/or periurethral striated muscle. Detrusor sphincter dyssynergia may involve striated or smooth muscle.

There is no coordinating centre for the control of micturition in the sacral cord. If the spinal cord above the sacrum is damaged a new neural pathway for reflex voiding comes into play. Activation of this reflex results in uncoordinated micturition.

The long routed micturition reflex is under the control of a variety of higher centres. The pathways involved are poorly understood. In childhood, intermittent involuntary contractions periodically empty the bladder. Continence requires that bladder contractions can be inhibited or facilitated to suit social circumstances. During childhood most people acquire the ability to inhibit bladder contraction. This allows bladder emptying to occur at a socially convenient time in an appropriate location. In addition, if we know that micturition is going to be inconvenient in the next few hours, we can prophylactically empty our bladder long before we have the urge to void.

The main centre responsible for the cortical control of micturition lies in the anteromedial part of the frontal lobe. Although it is generally believed that this area has an inhibitory effect on the micturition reflex it has been argued that this is a facilitatory area. Thus it is postulated that incontinence results from pathological stimulation of a facilitatory area rather than as a result of damage to an inhibitory area. The detrusor motor nucleus is thought to receive afferents from the basal ganglia, the cerebellum, the septal region and the anterior hypothalamus. The superior part of the pre- and post-central gyri is involved in the control of the striated muscles of the pelvic floor and the rhabdosphincter.

The physiology of micturition

Our understanding of the physiology of the lower urinary tract is incomplete, and aspects of the normal functioning of the bladder and urethra remains controversial. Some of these, such as the function of the sympathetic nervous system, innervation of the rhabdosphincter and the effect of cortical control on the long routed micturition reflex have already been referred to.

Functionally the lower urinary tract consists of the bladder and a 'sphincter'. There is, however, no discrete sphincter. The bladder neck and the proximal urethra act as the sphincteric mechanism.

There are two phases to lower urinary tract function—the filling phase and micturition. In a normal filling phase the bladder is able to accommodate a large volume of urine at low pressure, sensation is normal, there is no reflux of urine up the ureters, no leakage of urine from the bladder even under stress conditions and no involuntary bladder contractions.

Bladder function

As the bladder fills there is a small rise in intravesical pressure (Fig. 3) of less than 15 cmH$_2$O. Initially this is because the empty bladder is like a collapsed sac; it can fill to a certain level before any stretch is applied to the bladder wall. Once it starts to be stretched the ability of the bladder to accommodate increasing volumes of urine with little rise in intravesical pressure is due to the viscoelastic properties of its smooth muscle and connective tissue. The

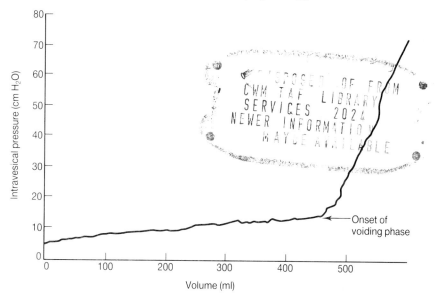

Figure 3 Filling cystometry.

response of the detrusor to stretch is referred to as its 'tone'. This is due to its inherent physical properties and is not directly affected by its nerve supply. The influence of the nervous system on the bladder is to control the micturition reflex. The nervous system affects bladder tone indirectly. Bladder tone is affected by the degree of stretching. Over-stretching leads to hypotonicity and lack of stretch to hypertonicity. The micturition reflex normally determines the degree of stretch of the muscle and thus indirectly affects bladder tone. The physical nature of the bladder wall may be affected by changes such as fibrosis.

The bladder fills at a rate of about 1 ml per minute. As it fills, afferent activity from stretch receptors increases. At a certain threshold level, which varies from person to person, this afferent activity will impinge on consciousness. The normal bladder capacity is around 500 ml. Males void at a pressure of 40–50 cmH$_2$O and a maximum flow rate of 30–40 ml per second. Females void at a pressure of 30–40 cmH$_2$O and a maximum flow rate of 40–50 ml per second. Normally there are no bladder contractions during filling. Voiding is usually deferred until a suitable time and site are found. This ability to defer voiding varies from individual to individual and may be altered by factors such as anxiety.

The intramural ureter passes through the bladder wall obliquely. This helps prevent vesicoureteric reflux because the intramural ureter is compressed as the bladder is stretched. During voiding, contraction of the bladder pulls the ureters downwards and medially. As the proximal end of the intramural ureter is fixed this results in lengthening of the intramural ureter and thus increases the resistance to retrograde flow.

The way in which voiding is initiated is unknown. Detrusor contraction is preceded by a drop in intraurethral pressure due to relaxation of the striated muscles of the urethra and pelvis floor. The mechanism of bladder neck opening is controversial. It is unknown whether it is an active or passive phenomenon. Voiding of urine occurs when the pressure difference between the bladder and urethra can overcome the elastic resistance of the urethra. Some women can void normally without a demonstrable rise in detrusor pressure.

At the end of micturition the striated muscles of the pelvic floor contract. This leads to interruption of urine flow at the level of the mid-urethra in the female. There is then 'milking back' of urine from the urethra to the bladder. If these striated muscles are contracted during micturition the interruption of urine flow results in a temporary rise in intravesical pressure as the detrusor contracts against a closed urethra. This results in reflex inhibition of the detrusor contraction and is the mechanism responsible for the voluntary cessation of micturition.

Urethral function

During the filling phase the pressure in the urethra exceeds the intravesical pressure. The difference between the urethral pressure and the intravesical pressure is referred to as the urethral closure pressure. The length of the urethra along which the urethral pressure exceeds the bladder pressure in the resting state is referred to as the functional urethral length. This is more important than the anatomical urethral length. Patients with a shortened anatomical length can remain continent.

The resting pressure in the urethra results from the action of the smooth muscle, the striated muscle, the elastic tension of the urethral connective tissue and the turgor of the blood vessels in the urethra. There is debate concerning the relative contribution made by each of these to urethral pressure. The vascular and connective tissue components are said to provide 30 per cent of the force, the smooth muscle 40 per cent and the striated muscle the remaining 30 per cent. The effect of the striated muscle is localized being maximal at the mid-point of the urethra in the female. It is in this area that intraurethral pressure is at its highest. The effect of the other components is more evenly distributed.

The increase in urethral closure pressure during bladder filling results from activity in both the smooth and striated muscles. It is mediated by a reflex with both the afferent and efferent limbs in the pelvic nerves. The urethra provides a water-tight seal. There is complete apposition of the rich folds of the urethral mucosa. The tension exerted by the smooth and striated muscle has to be exerted on a soft inner layer which is capable of being compressed. The lumen of the urethra is obliterated by this water-tight seal referred to as the mucosal seal mechanism.

In the standing position the base of the bladder is horizontal. The urethra and the trigone form an angle of less than 100 degrees. The urethral axis to the vertical does not exceed 30 degrees. During straining the normal bladder base remains horizontal but may descend by up to 1.5 cm. The urethra is fixed so that the bladder neck appears as a valve or kink.

The sphincter mechanism has to maintain the pressure difference between the urethra and the bladder under the stress of raised intra-abdominal pressure. It does this by virtue of the fact that the proximal urethra is an intra-abdominal organ. Pressure rises transmitted to the bladder are also transmitted to the proximal urethra thus maintaining the pressure differential. The pressure differential may increase during stress due to reflex increased activity in the pelvic floor muscles.

Age-related changes

With increasing age, bladder capacity, the ability to defer voiding and urinary flow rates diminish in both sexes. There is a small rise in the post-voiding residual but usually to no more than 50 ml. There is also an increase in the amount of urine formed and excreted at night. This occurs in the healthy elderly and is not confined to those with cardiac failure, renal disease or prostatic outflow obstruction. In females there is a reduction in urethral length and the maximal urethral closure pressure. Anatomically there is a relative decrease in the amount of urethral skeletal muscle and vascular tissue and a relative increase in the amount of connective tissue.

References

Andrew J, Nathan PW. Lesions of the anterior frontal lobes and disturbances of micturition and defaecation. *Brain* 1964; **87:** 234–265.

Gosling JA, Dixon JS. The structure and innervation of smooth muscle in the wall of the bladder neck and proximal urethra. *Br. J. Urol.* 1975; **47:** 549–558.

Gosling JA, Dixon JS, Lendon RG. The autonomic innervation of the human male and female bladder neck and proximal urethra. *J. Urol.* 1977; **118:** 302–305.

Juenemann, KP, Lue TF, Schmidt A, Tanagho EA. Clinical significance of sacral and pudendal nerve anatomy. *J. Urol.* 1988; **139:** 74–80.

Tanagho EA, Miller ER, Meyers FH, Corbett RK. Observations on the dynamics of the bladder neck. *Br. J. Urol.* 1966; **38:** 72–84.

Tang PC, Ruch TC. Non-neurogenic basis of bladder tonus. *Am. J. Physiol.* 1955; **181:** 249–257.

Vodusek DB, Keith Light J. The motor nerve supply of the external urethral sphincter muscles: an electrophysiological study. *Neurourol. Urodynam.* 1983; **2:** 193–200.

Chapter 2 _____

The pathophysiology of urinary incontinence

The International Continence Society defines urinary incontinence as a condition in which involuntary loss of urine is a social or hygienic problem and is objectively demonstrable. Different pathophysiological mechanisms can lead to incontinence. Table 1 lists some of the important causes.

Table 1 Urinary incontinence in the elderly

Transient
Toxic confusional state
Urinary tract infection
Faecal impaction
Drugs (e.g. diuretics, sedatives)

Established
Over-active detrusor
   detrusor hyperreflexia
   idiopathic detrusor instability
   obstructive detrusor instability
Genuine stress incontinence
Sensory urge incontinence
Overflow incontinence
Unstable urethra
Fistulae
Functional (e.g. depression, dementia, immobility)
Post-prostatectomy incontinence
Combination of factors

Urinary incontinence is divided into transient and established incontinence. This book is concerned primarily with the causes and management of established urinary incontinence.

Transient urinary incontinence

Transient incontinence of urine in the elderly usually occurs in association with a toxic confusional state. It is presumed that the patient loses awareness of the need to void at an appropriate time and an appropriate place. The incontinence can be expected to improve as the confusion resolves.

Urinary tract infection may lead to urinary incontinence. Infection may cause a toxic confusional state or may lead to sensory urge incontinence. Sensory urgency is discussed later. In patients with established urinary incontinence, infection of the lower urinary tract may be a complication of the pathophysiological mechanism leading to the incontinence. The presence of infection and incontinence does not necessarily mean that the incontinence is secondary to the infection. In established incontinence it is probable that both are secondary to the same underlying disorder.

Impaired mobility and various drugs, for example sedatives or diuretics, are also associated with transient incontinence. In some patients these are precipitating or aggravating factors rather than the primary problem. How faecal impaction causes incontinence is unclear. However, correction of faecal impaction may cure urinary incontinence as well as faecal incontinence.

Transient incontinence is said to account for about a third of incontinence among the elderly dwelling in the community and for half of the incontinence seen in acutely ill elderly patients admitted to hospital.

Established incontinence

The commonest causes of established urinary incontinence in the elderly are the over-active detrusor and genuine stress incontinence. Particular emphasis is placed on these conditions in the following discussions.

Over-active detrusor function

This term refers to involuntary detrusor contractions (Fig. 4). These contrac-

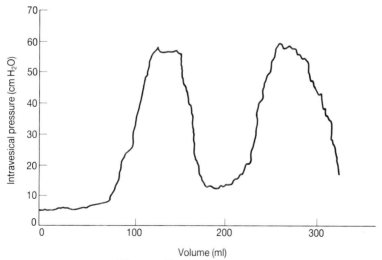

Figure 4 Detrusor instability.

tions, which the patient cannot suppress, may occur spontaneously during bladder filling or may be provoked by acts which raise intra-abdominal pressure. They may or may not be associated with urine loss. When detrusor over-activity is secondary to dysfunction of the neural control of the bladder the term detrusor hyperreflexia is used. In the absence of an identifiable neurological disorder the term unstable detrusor is used.

The unstable detrusor and detrusor hyperreflexia are urodynamic diagnoses. The diagnosis used to require the demonstration of a pressure rise of greater than 15 cm of water during filling cystometry or on the provocative testing of coughing, passive pressure changes, catheter withdrawal or coughing while standing. This choice of 15 cm of water as the cut-off point before unstable contractions could be diagnosed was somewhat arbitrary. The International Continence Society no longer recognizes any specific value as being essential to make the diagnosis. It is implicit in the International Continence Society's definition of what constitutes an unstable contraction that the pressure rise should be phasic. The contraction should be followed by some degree of relaxation.

Where a gradual increase in pressure is seen throughout filling the term low-compliance bladder is used. This is often seen in patients with neuropathic bladder disorders. It is important because its presence in these patients is associated with upper tract complications. The mechanism is unclear. It may be neurally mediated, though recent studies suggest that it is due to an increased amount of connective tissue in the bladder wall. Low compliance will also be found in the shrunken fibrotic bladders of patients with interstitial cystitis, tuberculous cystitis or those who have had radiotherapy. During cystometry a transient rise in pressure indicates an involuntary contraction. A sustained pressure rise may be due to low compliance or a sustained contraction. These involuntary contractions have been shown to be real and not just artefacts due to the unphysiological procedure of cystometry.

Although they may be asymptomatic, involuntary contractions can result in the symptoms of urinary frequency, nocturia, urgency, urge incontinence and stress incontinence. The frequency and nocturia occur because the bladder typically contracts at a lower volume than normal. This is not invariably the case. Some diabetics show unstable activity generated by bladder filling which require a large urinary volume to provoke the response. Frequency is defined as voiding more than seven times per day or more than two-hourly. Most people over the age of 60 have to pass urine at least once during the night. A further visit to the toilet can be added for each further decade before nocturia is regarded as abnormal. It is only at the onset of the detrusor contraction, or occasionally just at the time of urethral urinary flow, that the patient is aware of the bladder contraction. If the patient is unable to get to the toilet in time the sensation of urgency gives way to urge incontinence. Patients with neurological disorders may lose urine without any warning. This is referred to as reflex incontinence. It may also occur in patients with involuntary urethral relaxation.

The involuntary loss of urine associated with a strong desire to void is called urge incontinence. Urgency associated with an over-active detrusor is referred to as motor urgency. Urgency and urge incontinence may also occur in hypersensitive bladder conditions, when they are referred to as sensory urgency and sensory urge incontinence. Although incontinence is common in patients with motor urgency it is much less common in those with sensory urgency. The patient with sensory urgency has a strong desire to void but has not lost control over his or her bladder. If such patients are incontinent it is because they choose to wet themselves rather than tolerate the sensation of urgency until the time and place are appropriate for micturition.

If involuntary contractions are precipitated by a rise in intra-abdominal pressure the patient may complain of stress incontinence. Where this is due to an involuntary detrusor contraction the volume lost is often large and there may be a short delay between the stimulus and the loss of urine. If the volume of urine lost is small the patient may report a poor urinary stream. Urinary flow rates are proportional to the volume voided up to a total of 300 ml. Some patients with detrusor instability may persistently pass volumes of urine less than this.

Between the ages of 10 and 30 years around 10–15 per cent of the population are believed to have an over-active detrusor. The prevalence rises with age. It has been shown to be present in up to 50 per cent of elderly men and 30 per cent of elderly women investigated in urodynamic units.

The causes of detrusor hyperreflexia will be considered later in this chapter. The unstable detrusor may be obstructive or idiopathic. Outflow obstruction is common in elderly men where it is usually due to prostatic hyperplasia. Fifty per cent of men with significant outflow tract obstruction have unstable bladders. The occurrence of bladder instability correlates with the degree of outflow obstruction. There is, however, no correlation between the severity of the obstruction and the degree of instability. With surgical relief of the outflow obstruction around two-thirds of the patients will regain continence as the detrusor instability resolves. This usually takes up to six months to occur. In some patients it may be a year before continence is restored. The number of men with persistent instability after relief of outflow obstruction approximates to the number of women of the same age who have detrusor instability. Outflow obstruction is rare in women and is not associated with detrusor instability. By definition the cause of idiopathic detrusor instability is unknown. In younger age groups it is usually considered to be a psychosomatic disorder. It has been suggested that many older patients without obvious outflow obstruction or overt neurological disease have subclinical cerebral damage as the cause of their instability.

The pathophysiological mechanism leading to the unstable detrusor is unknown. Experimental evidence suggests substantial differences between idiopathic and obstructive instability. In obstructive instability the detrusor shows reduced sensitivity to electrical stimulation of its nerve supply and increased sensitivity to stimulation by acetylcholine and to direct electrical stimulation of the muscle itself. In idiopathic instability the detrusor shows increased sensitivity to stimulation of its nerve supply and to acetylcholine, and response to direct electrical stimulation is normal. These abnormalities are compatible with a membrane potential which is more unstable than normal, possibly due to loss of an inhibitory neurotransmitter. It has been suggested that idiopathic instability results from a disorder of intrinsic inhibition. One suggestion for the deficient inhibitory neurotransmitter is vasoactive intestinal polypeptide. Nerves containing vasoactive intestinal polypeptide have been identified in the normal bladder. A reduction of vasoactive intestinal polypeptide concentrations has been found in the bladders of patients with idiopathic detrusor instability.

Resnick and Yalla have recently identified a condition they call detrusor hyperactivity with impaired contractility (DHIC), in which involuntary bladder contractions show a slow rate of rise of detrusor pressure and expel less than half the volume of urine in the bladder. Other workers have been unable to confirm this. It is also worth mentioning here the condition referred to as handwashing incontinence. This occurs on washing hands in cold water, washing clothes, hearing the sound of running water and going outside from a warm room into a cold environment. It is usually due to involuntary detrusor contractions and is said to affect about 15 per cent of the over 60s.

Genuine stress incontinence

Stress incontinence may be a symptom or a sign. It is important to remember that the symptom or sign of stress incontinence may be found not only in patients with genuine stress incontinence but also in patients with detrusor instability, detrusor hyperreflexia, urethral instability or overflow incontinence. The International Continence Society defines genuine stress incontinence as a condition in which there is involuntary loss of urine when the intravesical pressure exceeds the maximum urethral pressure due to elevation of intra-abdominal pressure and in the absence of detrusor contraction (Fig. 5).

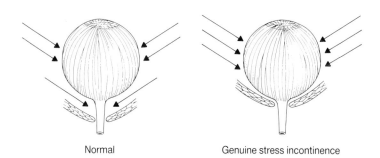

Normal   Genuine stress incontinence

Figure 5 Raised intra-abdominal pressure.

Genuine stress incontinence is usually due to failure of the anatomical support of the bladder and urethra. Among the structures supporting the bladder neck are the posterior pubourethral ligaments, the pubocervical fascia and the levator ani muscle. Childbirth and post-menopausal atrophy due to oestrogen deficiency are considered contributory to the failure of anatomical support. Because of defects in the support of the bladder neck and proximal urethra the urethra becomes an extra-abdominal organ either at rest or when intra-abdominal pressure is raised. As a result raised intra-abdominal pressure is transmitted to the bladder raising intravesical pressure but is not transmitted efficiently to the proximal urethra. There is a transient reversal of the pressure gradient with intravesical pressure now exceeding intraurethral pressure. This results in urine loss. The significance of impaired pressure transmission is dependent on the magnitude of the urethral closure pressure. The greater the closure pressure the greater the degree of inefficient transmission that can be tolerated before incontinence results. The loss of anatomical support in addition to allowing downward and posterior rotational movement of the bladder neck and proximal urethra, places the urethra in a dependent position with respect to the bladder neck. It also results in loss of the kinking mechanism that occurs between the bladder neck and urethra. These changes may result in the angle between the urethral axis and the vertical increasing to greater than 30 degrees and the urethrotrigonal angle increasing to greater than 100 degrees. Although these changes in angle are associated with genuine stress incontinence they are not pathognomonic. Some women have abnormal angles but remain continent.

In the situation just described the sphincter mechanism itself is normal and can maintain a watertight seal. Incontinence occurs because the sphincter mechanism is in an abnormal position when intra-abdominal pressure rises. In some patients with genuine stress incontinence the sphincter mechanism can no longer maintain a watertight seal. This is referred to as Type III stress incontinence. In this condition incontinence occurs on the slightest provocation. It usually occurs in patients who have had previous surgery for stress incontinence. The resultant scarring leads to a rigid urethra, preventing proper compression of the urethra and thus efficient transmission of intra-abdominal pressure. Rarely the condition may result from damage to the sympathetic supply to the urethra. This may occur secondary to aortic surgery, sympathectomy, radical perineal surgery or spinal cord damage. The importance of this condition is that it will not respond to the usual types of surgery for genuine stress incontinence. These are aimed at restoring the bladder neck and urethra to their normal anatomical position. Correction of the compression defect requires the use of urethral sling procedures, Teflon injections or an artificial sphincter.

Genuine stress incontinence is usually divided into five types.

Type 0 The patient gives a history of stress incontinence but this cannot be demonstrated on testing. The bladder neck is closed and lies above the superior markings of the pubic symphysis.

Type I The bladder neck is closed at rest and lies above the inferior margin of the pubic symphysis. During stress the bladder neck descends less than 2 cm.

Type IIa As Type I except that the bladder neck descends more than 2 cm during stress.

Type IIb Though closed at rest, the bladder neck lies below the inferior margin of the pubic symphysis.

Type III The bladder neck and proximal urethra are open at rest. Urine leakage is either gravitational or occurs on minimal stress.

Although stress incontinence is the expected symptom in patients with genuine stress incontinence, they may also have other lower urinary tract symptoms including urinary frequency, nocturia, urgency and urge incontinence.

Stress incontinence in the male

Stress incontinence is a much rarer symptom in the male. It most commonly results from sphincter damage at prostatic resection. Fortunately it occurs in less than 1 per cent of those who have transurethral resection of the prostate (TURP). It is more common after radical prostatectomy, affecting 5–10 per cent of patients. Post-prostatectomy incontinence may also be due to persistent detrusor instability. Where surgery is performed for benign prostatic hyperplasia post-surgical incontinence is usually due to detrusor instability. After radical prostatectomy for adenocarcinoma of the prostrate, sphincteric damage is the commonest cause. Stress incontinence in the male may also be a consequence of severe pelvic trauma or, more rarely, may result from damage to the nerve supply of the proximal urethra.

The unstable urethra

This is a poorly understood condition in which there are fluctuations in urethral pressure of greater than 15 cm of water. It can be associated with a variety of lower urinary tract symptoms including stress incontinence. Some of these patients are unable to initiate voiding voluntarily. It is a condition which affects mainly young women in whom no objective urological or neurological abnormality can be found. The condition may also be found in some patients with spinal injury.

Sensory urgency

Patients with sensory urgency suffer suprapubic discomfort and a constant urge to void. The condition may be idiopathic (another poorly understood disorder) or secondary to a variety of conditions including interstitial cystitis, lower urinary tract infection, bladder calculi, bladder neoplasms or radiation damage. Patients usually complain of frequency and nocturia in addition to urgency. As already mentioned, incontinence is less common in patients with sensory urgency than in patients with motor urgency.

Fistulae

Fistulae usually lead to constant urinary leakage. In developed countries the commonest cause of a vesicovaginal fistula is gynaecological surgery, especially hysterectomy. Fistulae can also result from damage during urological surgery, bowel surgery and from radiotherapy to pelvic malignancy. In the last case the fistula may not occur until 20 years after the course of radiotherapy. Neoplastic involvement of the bladder and urethra can also lead to fistula formation. In the developing world the commonest cause of a vesicovaginal fistula is obstetric trauma. Fistulae usually present as continuous diurnal and nocturnal incontinence.

Functional incontinence

This refers to the situation where the patient is incontinent despite a normally functioning lower urinary tract. This may occur in depression where the patient may be unconcerned about maintaining continence. It may also occur in some cognitively impaired patients who are unaware of the social requirement to maintain continence.

Voiding dysfunction

The International Continence Society defines overflow incontinence as any loss of urine associated with over-distention of the bladder. This may or may not be associated with a detrusor contraction. These patients typically have frequent or almost continuous loss of urine. The conditions leading to voiding dysfunction can be divided into those causing bladder outlet obstruction and those leading to the under-active detrusor.

Under-active detrusor function may have myogenic, neurogenic or psychogenic causes. A bladder which does not contract is referred to as a non-contractile detrusor. When this under-activity is due to an abnormality of the neural control of the bladder the condition is called detrusor areflexia. Lesions leading to detrusor areflexia are usually associated with other neurological abnormalities on clinical examination. The patient may be found to have lax anal tone on rectal examination, impaired perianal sensation, inability to contract voluntarily the external sphincter or an absent bulbo-cavernous reflex. At present urodynamic investigations cannot separate myogenic, psychogenic and neurogenic causes of an under-active detrusor. Recognition of appropriate neurological abnormalities is required before a diagnosis of detrusor areflexia can be made.

In females voiding disorders are very difficult to diagnose clinically. Few females with symptoms suggestive of voiding dysfunction prove to have a voiding disorder. Among those with voiding disorders frequency and urgency are the commonest symptoms. Only in females with urinary retention can the diagnosis be made with certainty. This problem will be reviewed later as will the causes of detrusor areflexia. One of the commonest causes of detrusor under-activity is the large, poorly contracting female bladder of unknown aetiology. This condition is commoner than the hypocontractile hyposensitive bladder which results from neurological lesions.

Outlet obstruction is common in elderly males where it is usually due to benign prostatic hypertrophy. Other causes include prostatic carcinoma, urethral stricture, faecal impaction, detrusor sphincter dyssynergia and the use of various drugs, such as anticholinergics, tricyclic antidepressants and phenothiazines. Although symptoms suggestive of voiding dysfunction are common in females, bladder outlet obstruction is much rarer in females than in males. With the obvious exception of prostatic lesions, it may result from any of the causes listed above. It may also be caused by the urethral distortion or kinking which can occur in patients with a uterovaginal prolapse or a large cystocele. Very rarely uterine fibroids or a large ovarian cyst may cause urethral compression.

Neuropathic bladder disorders

The term neuropathic bladder disorder is applied when dysfunction of the lower urinary tract results from injury to, or disease of, its neuronal control (Fig. 6). No neurological disorders affects the bladder alone. It is rare for a

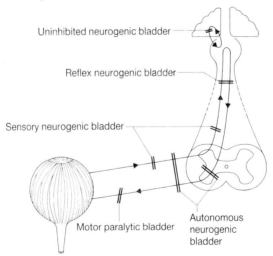

Uninhibited neurogenic bladder

Reflex neurogenic bladder

Sensory neurogenic bladder

Motor paralytic bladder

Autonomous neurogenic bladder

Figure 6 Neuropathic bladder disorders.

disease of the nervous system to manifest itself solely with urinary symptoms. Other neurological abnormalities, however, may only be detected after a careful neurological examination. A variety of different systems have been used to classify neuropathic bladder disorders. All have their limitations. One of the more useful systems divides neuropathic bladder disorders as follows: uninhibited; reflex neurogenic; autonomous neurogenic; sensory neurogenic; and motor paralytic.

Uninhibited neurogenic bladder

This results from damage to the corticoregulatory tract. The lesion may be at any level above the sacral segments of the spinal cord. It is associated with detrusor hyperreflexia. Sensation is usually normal and there is no significant residual urine. The patient can usually initiate voiding providing he or she can store sufficient urine before the onset of an involuntary contraction. Among the disorders associated with the uninhibited neuropathic bladder are cerebrovascular disease, Alzheimer's disease, tumours, multiple sclerosis, Parkinson's disease and cerebellar lesions. It may also result from an incomplete spinal cord lesion.

Reflex neurogenic bladder

This results from complete suprasacral interruption of the fibres to and from the detrusor motor nucleus in the brainstem. In addition to detrusor hyperreflexia there is absent vesical sensation, inability to initiate a voluntary detrusor contraction and a large residual urine due to detrusor sphincter dyssynergia. This disorder may occur after traumatic spinal cord injury or as a result of multiple sclerosis, transverse myelitis, spinal cord tumour, vascular lesions or cervical radiculopathy.

Autonomous neurogenic bladder

This results either from total destruction of the second to fourth sacral segments of the spinal cord or from extensive injury to both the afferent and efferent nerve supply of the bladder. There is absent sensation from the bladder and the patient cannot initiate a voluntary contraction. The amount of residual urine present depends upon the ability of the patient to increase intravesical pressure by straining and on the outflow resistance. The resistance offered by the sphincter mechanism depends on the intactness of its nerve supply. These patients may have weak poorly sustained detrusor contractions known as autonomous contractions. Voiding is incomplete because the bladder neck remains competent. Patients with sacral cord lesions may develop a low-compliance bladder with the associated dangers of upper tract deteriorations. Patients with an autonomous neurogenic bladder may have overflow or stress incontinence. This type of lesion can result from tumours, trauma or multiple sclerosis.

Sensory neurogenic bladder

This occurs when the sensory afferents from the bladder to the brainstem are damaged either in the peripheral nerves or in the sensory afferent tracts in the spinal cord. The patient loses the desire to void. Unless voiding is initiated out of habit, bladder over-distension occurs with resultant overflow incontinence. Once the bladder is over-distended, for whatever reason, its contractility will diminish. This type of neuropathic bladder may be found in patients with diabetes mellitus, tabes dorsalis or pernicious anaemia.

Motor paralytic bladder

This occurs when the efferent parasympathetic supply to the bladder is damaged. Although sensation is normal the patient cannot voluntarily initiate micturition. Bladder over-distension occurs leading to overflow incontinence. This disorder results from surgical damage, severe pelvic fracture, poliomyelitis or herpes zoster infection. A motor paralytic bladder is estimated to occur in around 8 per cent of patients after abdominoperineal resection for rectal carcinoma.

Although this classification system allows gross localization of the neurological lesion producing lower urinary tract dysfunction, many patients do not fit neatly into one of the above categories. This is because they have mixed or incomplete lesions. In addition, the pattern of abnormality found may be altered by secondary changes which occur in the bladder, such as over-distension or re-innervation. Nor does the classification system take account of associated sphincter function. For example, around two-thirds of patients with a reflex neurogenic bladder will have a detrusor sphincter dyssynergia.

Lesions affecting the cerebral cortex are expected to result in detrusor hyperreflexia. Lesions affecting the suprasacral spinal cord are expected to lead to detrusor hyperreflexia with striated sphincter dyssynergia. If the lesion is above the sixth thoracic level, smooth sphincter dyssynergia may also occur. Sacral cord lesions are expected to be associated with detrusor areflexia with a competent but non-relaxing smooth sphincter and a striated sphincter which is no longer under voluntary control. These expectations are based on the assumption that lesions are complete and are localized to one area. A minority of patients with high spinal cord lesions will be found to have detrusor areflexia. The majority of these will have evidence of a sacral cord lesion on clinical examination. The detrusor areflexia is presumed to be due to a coincidental sacral cord lesion. Similarly, some patients with sacral cord lesions have detrusor hyperreflexia. Although most patients will have the lower urinary tract dysfunction that is expected on the basis of the general neurological examination, this is not always the case. Management should be based on urodynamic findings rather than on assumptions made from the neurological findings.

Diseases causing neuropathic bladder dysfunction

Among the more common lesions causing neuropathic bladder dysfunction in the elderly are: cerebrovascular disease; Parkinson's disease; diabetes mellitus; multiple sclerosis; chronic brain failure; and spinal cord trauma.

Cerebrovascular disease
Cerebrovascular disease usually leads to an unhibited neuropathic bladder with detrusor hyperreflexia. Detrusor sphincter dyssynergia is rare in these patients. Lesions in both hemispheres are associated with bladder dysfunction. It is not as yet known if incontinence is more common, as has been suggested, in dominant hemisphere lesions. In addition to causing an uninhibited neuropathic bladder, cerebrovascular disease may lead to impaired mobility and communication problems. These in turn act as aggravating factors. For the same reasons patients with a pre-existing unstable detrusor may have urinary urgency converted to urge incontinence because they are no longer able to reach the toilet in time. The situation may be further aggravated by confusion or depression. The same problem may arise in other neurological disorders, such as multiple sclerosis and Parkinson's disease, which as well as causing detrusor hyperreflexia also affect mobility, communication and manual dexterity. Although incontinence is common in the early stages of a stroke it is usually transient. Only 15–30 per cent of survivors remain incontinent six months following the stroke. Incontinence has a useful prognostic value in patients who have had a stroke. Only 3 per cent of those who are continent on day 1 of the stroke will die within the first month. Those incontinent after a stroke who regain normal bladder function within the first month have a greater than 80 per cent chance of returning to the community within six months.

Parkinson's disease
The basal ganglia are thought to exert an inhibitory action on the detrusor motor nucleus in the pons. Parkinson's disease is thus usually associated with an uninhibited neurogenic bladder. The anticholinergic medication these patients may receive can cause detrusor under-activity. Some patients with Parkinson's disease show sphincter bradykinesia. The pelvic floor muscles are slow to relax at the onset of a detrusor contraction. This abnormality appears to be peculiar to parkinsonian patients.

Diabetes mellitus
Lower urinary tract dysfunction due to autonomic neuropathy is relatively rare in diabetics. It correlates with the severity of the diabetes rather than its duration. There is early loss of sensation and the development of a sensory neurogenic bladder. There is nearly always an associated sensory peripheral neuropathy. Diabetics may also demonstrate detrusor hyperreflexia which requires a large urinary volume to provoke the response.

Multiple sclerosis
Lower urinary tract symptoms are common in multiple sclerosis with over 50 per cent of patients affected. Half of the remaining patients who have no urinary symptoms will be found to have abnormalities on urodynamic testing.

As with diabetes mellitus, the severity of urinary symptoms correlates with the degree of disability but not with the duration of the disease. Urinary symptoms are the sole presenting feature in less than 2 per cent of cases. They form part of the initial symptom complex in about 12 per cent of patients. Three patterns of neuropathic bladder dysfunction are recognized. Two-thirds of symptomatic patients have detrusor hyperreflexia. Half of these will have detrusor sphincter dyssynergia. Around a quarter of symptomatic patients are found to have detrusor areflexia. Unlike the neurological symptoms the urinary symptoms rarely remit spontaneously. Ultimately around 5 per cent of patients die of urinary tract complications.

Chronic brain failure
Chronic brain failure most commonly due to senile dementia of the Alzheimer's type is associated with an uninhibited neurogenic bladder. Little is known concerning the prevalence of incontinence in non-institutionalized patients with dementia. Nor is it known whether incontinence is commoner or occurs earlier in multi-infarct dementia or Alzheimer's disease. Incontinence in these patients may be due to lack of awareness of the need to void in an appropriate setting. Incontinence due to detrusor hyperreflexia may be aggravated by inability to locate the toilet.

Spinal cord trauma
Traumatic lesions to the spinal cord are in general a problem of younger age groups. Urinary tract dysfunction remains the main cause of morbidity and mortality in these patients, renal impairment being a consequence of impaired renal drainage, infection and amyloid disease. Damage to the sacral cord or cauda equina results in an autonomous neurogenic bladder. The detrusor is acontractile. After a few days or weeks the bladder neck may become increasingly incompetent. Why this occurs is unknown. One consequence of this is that the patient may be able to void by straining or by manual compression. Initially patients with suprasacral lesions will be in spinal shock and will also have an acontractile bladder. Most later develop detrusor hyperreflexia but this may take weeks or months to develop. It may be associated with detrusor sphincter dyssynergia. Patients with suprasacral lesions may continue to have incomplete bladder emptying. This has two causes: the development of detrusor sphincter dyssynergia and the fact that involuntary detrusor contractions are often poorly sustained. Although the management of incontinence is the subject of later chapters, a number of points regarding the treatment of patients with traumatic spinal cord lesions are appropriately mentioned here. The primary aim of management is the preservation of renal function rather than the restoration of continence. Initial management is usually by intermittent self-catheterization. This technique is described later. It is particularly useful in those with an acontractile bladder. In those who later develop detrusor hyperreflexia, bladder emptying is promoted by tapping the suprapubic area for around 20 seconds in an

attempt to induce a detrusor contraction. This is followed by suprapubic abdominal compression. Between voids male patients will usually use a condom catheter. The alternatives are to continue with intermittent self-catheterization combined with the use of drug therapy to reduce the degree of detrusor hyperreflexia, or the use of a permanent indwelling catheter. Many male patients find intermittent self-catheterization unacceptable. It may also fail because of loss of hand function or if the patient continues to have episodes of incontinence between catheterizations. In practice most of the elderly will require an indwelling catheter.

The development of detrusor sphincter dyssynergia in patients with supra-sacral lesions may lead to an elevated residual urine, infection, vesicoureteric reflux and hydronephrosis. These patients require an endoscopic external urethral sphincterotomy. Patients with cervical and high thoracic cord lesions may develop autonomic dysreflexia. This is usually triggered by a distended bladder, for example, if a catheter becomes blocked. It is due to reflex sympathetic over-activity and leads to vasoconstriction and hypertension. Baroreceptor stimulation then leads to reflex bradycardia but cannot lead to reflex vasodilatation as the spinal cord tracts involved are blocked. Symptoms include headaches, sweating and flushing. Treatment involves relief of the bladder distension and, if necessary, the use of hypotensive agents.

Many other neurological diseases can give rise to the neuropathic bladder. Among these are normal pressure hydrocephalus, lumbar spondylosis, inter-vertebral disc prolapse, transverse myelitis, tumours, vascular lesions of the spinal cord, tabes dorsalis, herpes zoster and arachnoiditis.

Urinary incontinence in the elderly

There have been few series of urodynamic studies in non-incontinent elderly people. In one study nearly half of the patients had evidence of neurological disease. Overall, half those studied had an over-active detrusor. In a second study nearly two-thousand elderly people living in the community were randomly selected and offered free urodynamic studies. Less than 10 per cent accepted. As in the previous study there was a high prevalence of detrusor instability in these continent elderly subjects.

Urodynamic studies on elderly patients with established incontinence have shown that between 40 and 75 per cent have over-active detrusors. In contrast to studies in younger age groups, many of these elderly patients have an identifiable neurological lesion. Detrusor over-activity appears to be the commonest cause of established urinary incontinence in the elderly. Genuine stress incontinence is common among elderly females. Combined lesions may occur. Many elderly patients have at least two pathophysiological mechan-isms for their incontinence. Even where there is a single pathophysiological mechanisms it may be difficult to know which of two pathologies is causing it. An elderly man with an over-active detrusor may have Parkinson's disease and prostatic hyperplasia. It is difficult to be certain whether or not he has detrusor hyperreflexia or obstructive detrusor instability. This obviously has implications for management and this problem will be reviewed later.

In the elderly much more than in younger age groups, factors outside the lower urinary tract are often important in the aetiology, precipitation and worsening of incontinence. Factors such as the patient's cognitive state, mood and mobility should always be carefully assessed when attempting to identify the cause of an elderly patient's incontinence.

References

Blaivas JG, Bhimani G, Labib KB. Vesicourethral dysfunction in multiple sclerosis. *J. Urol.* 1979; **122:** 342–347.

Castleten CM, Duffin HM, Asher MJ. Clinical and urodynamic studies in 100 elderly incontinent patients. *Br. Med. J.* 1981; **282:** 1103–1105.

Cucchi A. Detrusor instability and bladder outflow obstruction. Evidence for a correlation between the severity of obstruction and the presence of instability. *Br. J. Urol.* 1988; **61:** 420–422.

Jones KW, Schoenberg HW. Comparisons of the incidence of bladder hyperreflexia in patients with benign prostatic hypertrophy and age-matched female controls. *J. Urol.* 1985; **133:** 425–426.

Kaplan SA, Chancellor MB, Blaivias JG. Bladder and sphincter behaviour in patients with spinal cord lesions. *J. Urol.* 1991; **146:** 113–117.

Khan Z, Hartenu, J, Yang WC, Melman A, Leiter E. Predictive correlation of urodynamic dysfunction and brain injury after cerebrovascular accident. *J. Urol.* 1981; **126:** 86–88.

Kinder RB, Mundy AR. Pathophysiology of idiopathic detrusor instability and detrusor hyperreflexia. *Br. J. Urol.* 1987; **60:** 509–515.

Pavlakis AJ, Siroky MB, Goldstein I, Krane RJ. Neurological findings in Parkinson's disease. *J. Urol.* 1983; **129:** 80–83.

Resnick N, Yalla S. *J.A.M.A.* 1987; **257:** 3076.

Wein AJ. Classification of neurogenic voiding dysfunction. *J. Urol.* 1981; **125:** 605–609.

Chapter 3 _____

Epidemiological and psychological aspects of incontinence

Epidemiology

There is wide variation in the reported prevalence of urinary incontinence in the elderly, especially in community studies. A number of explanations have been advanced to explain these discrepancies. Those who are incontinent may be more likely to reply to questionnaires on incontinence. Alternatively, under-reporting may arise because some of those surveyed are too embarrassed to acknowledge their incontinence. Where questions regarding continence are part of a wider survey, respondents may consider them unimportant. They may feel that it is reasonable to withhold what they consider to be embarrassing answers to unimportant questions. It is well-established that there is a higher than average prevalence of incontinence among those who are cognitively impaired. These patients are unlikely to reply to postal questionnaires. Where they are interviewed their replies are unlikely to be accurate.

Most of the variation between the different studies is probably due to the different definitions of incontinence used. Thomas and her co-workers found the prevalence of incontinence in the elderly to be 11.6 per cent in females and 6.9 per cent in males. They defined incontinence as the involuntary loss of urine on two or more occasions per month. Yarnell and St Leger defined incontinence as the involuntary loss of urine any time in the previous year. Not surprisingly, they found a higher prevalence of incontinence among the elderly than Thomas *et al*. In their study 17 per cent of women and 11 per cent of men were incontinent. In general, the studies to date have found an overall prevalence of incontinence in the elderly of between 12 and 15 per cent. Some have reported levels as high as 30 per cent. As well as having different definitions of incontinence, authors have also defined its severity in different ways. Allowing for this, most studies have found that between 3 and 7 per cent of the elderly suffer from 'frequent' urinary incontinence. All of these studies have shown that the prevalence of incontinence rises with age. They have also shown a marked sex difference, with women on average being affected twice as often as men.

In studies on the prevalence of incontinence in the community it has been found that 50–70 per cent of the incontinent elderly are unknown to the medical nursing or social services. This under-reporting occurs for a number of reasons. Some patients believe that incontinence is a normal consequence of ageing. Others are too embarrassed to acknowledge its existence. Patients may believe that nothing can be done about their incontinence or, alternatively, may fear being pressurized into having surgery if they report it. Not only does incontinence often go unreported but many of those who do seek professional help have been incontinent for a long time before reporting the problem.

As with studies on the prevalence of incontinence in the community, studies of incontinence among those in residential care have also asked different questions concerning its prevalence and severity. Early studies found that around 17 per cent of residents were incontinent of urine. More recent studies have found prevalence rates of around 30 per cent. The higher prevalence of incontinence among those in residential care is presumably related to their more advanced age and to the higher prevalence of physical and mental morbidity in this population. The change over time within the homes themselves is a reflection of the increasing level of dependency of those in residential care.

As might be expected, the prevalence of incontinence is higher still among those in nursing homes, continuing-care geriatric beds and continuing-care psychogeriatric beds. Around 50 per cent of patients in nursing homes, 70 per cent of patients in continuing-care geriatric beds and 80 per cent of patients in long-stay psychogeriatric wards are incontinent of urine. Many of those in institutional care who are incontinent of urine are also incontinent of faeces.

Psychological aspects of incontinence

The presence of urinary incontinence often results in significant psychological and social morbidity. The psychological impact of incontinence bears no relationship to its severity. A woman with mild stress incontinence may be severely distressed. Another with severe urge incontinence may be relatively unperturbed. It has been found that incontinence has little if any effect on the self-esteem of many older patients. This surprising finding may be because they perceive it to be a normal age-related phenomenon. Many are already significantly disabled in other ways. The addition of incontinence to their other disabilities has little further impact on their self-image.

Patients may deal with being incontinent by denial. An otherwise sensible patient may lie in soaking sheets adamantly denying that she has ever been incontinent. More often patients are embarrassed and ashamed. They attempt to hide all evidence of their incontinence. Their day becomes centred on the need to be near a toilet and this restricts their ability to socialize. Shame and embarrassment about soiled clothes, a uriniferous smell and fear of having an accident leads them to restrict their social interaction. A number of studies have confirmed that incontinent patients have reduced contact with others, restrict their social activities and are significantly more anxious and depressed. Patients with detrusor instability usually suffer greater psychological problems than those with genuine stress incontinence.

Younger patients in particular report sexual difficulties. This is commoner among those with detrusor instability than among those with genuine stress incontinence. Around half of all female patients attending for urodynamic studies report sexual difficulties related to their incontinence. A quarter are incontinent during intercourse.

Psychological problems may contribute to the development of incontinence. Patients who are severely depressed may be so low in mood that they cease to take themselves to the toilet and appear unconcerned by the resultant incontinence, making no effort to change wet clothes or to move from wet chairs. It has been suggested that the idiopathic unstable detrusor is a psychosomatic problem. However, in these patients it remains impossible to separate cause and effect. We don't as yet know whether the high level of anxiety and depression among incontinent patients is a consequence of their being incontinent, or whether psychological factors are aetiologically important in the development of detrusor instability.

The response of others must also be considered. The development of incontinence increases the physical, psychological and financial burden of caring for frail and disabled relatives. It is often cited as a factor precipitating institutionalization. In residential homes continent residents often ostracize those who are incontinent. Care staff and nursing staff may develop negative feelings towards the incontinent. Caring for incontinent residents or patients is more time-consuming and may have a negative effect on staff morale. Care staff and nursing staff may respond to the development of incontinence in one of three ways. They may consider it an inevitable and unavoidable part of caring for the elderly. They may view it as deviant or bad behaviour. If properly trained they will look upon it as a medical and nursing problem requiring appropriate assessment and management.

The response of doctors to incontinent patients is often inadequate. It is not usually considered important. Despite its prevalence it is not included in many doctors' routine history taking. Because of their embarrassment patients rarely volunteer that they have a problem with urinary control. This increases the onus upon the doctor to ask the appropriate questions. When its presence is brought to the attention of medical staff by patients or nursing staff the problem is often ignored. Doctors, unless they have a special interest in the subject, tend to view incontinence as a nursing problem and thus not their responsibility.

References

Campbell AJ, Reinken J, McCosh L. Incontinence in the elderly: prevalence and prognosis, *Age Ageing* 1985; **14:** 65–70.

Hodkinson E, McCafferty FG, Scott JN, Stout RW. Disability and dependency in elderly people in residential and hospital care. *Age Ageing* 1988; **17:** 147–154.

Macauley AJ, Stern RS, Holmes DM, Stanton SL. Micturition and the mind: psychological factors in the aetiology and treatment of urinary symptoms in women. *Br. Med. J.* 1987; **294:** 540–543.

Norton PA, MacDonald LD, Sedgwick PM, Stanton SL. Distress and delay associated with urinary incontinence, frequency, and urgency in women. *Br. Med. J.* 1988; **297:** 1187–1189.

Thomas TM, Plymat KR, Blannin J, Meade TW. Prevalence of urinary incontinence. *Br. Med. J.* 1980; **281:** 1243–1245.

Tobin GW, Brocklehurst JC. The management of urinary incontinence in local authority residential homes for the elderly. *Age Ageing* 1986; **15:** 292–298.

Yarnell JWG, St Leger AS. The prevalence severity and factors associated with urinary incontinence in a random sample of the elderly. *Age Ageing* 1979; **8:** 81–85.

Chapter 4 _____

Diagnosis and the use of urodynamic investigations

It is an oft quoted maxim that the bladder is an unreliable witness. Because the different pathophysiological mechanisms producing urinary incontinence may lead to similar lower urinary tract symptoms, diagnoses based on clinical assessment alone are often inaccurate. Although urodynamic investigations are necessary for an accurate diagnosis they are not a prerequisite for the management of all incontinent patients. Their place in the management of the incontinent elderly is controversial. While it has been claimed that attempting to manage incontinent patients without prior urodynamic studies is analogous to treating a cardiac arrhythmia without first obtaining an ECG, most physicians in geriatric medicine manage their incontinent patients without prior recourse to urodynamic studies. The correct answer must lie between these extremes. This chapter reviews the problems involved in trying to arrive at a clinical diagnosis and describes some of the more common urodynamic investigations along with the indications for their use.

Assessment of the incontinent patient

Assessment of the incontinent patient starts with the history. In addition to noting the patient's age and sex, the history should include questions about duration of incontinence, frequency of incontinence and the volume of urine lost. Enquiry should be made into the presence of urinary frequency, nocturia, urgency, urge incontinence, stress incontinence and hesitancy, the character of the urinary stream, presence of terminal dribbling, need to strain when voiding, feelings of incomplete emptying after voiding, haematuria, dysuria, number and type of protective pads used, previous urological and gynaecological surgery, neurological history and medication.

Clinical examination should include examination of the abdomen looking for a palpable bladder. Patients should have a rectal examination looking for faecal impaction. The presence or absence of the anal reflex, the anal sphincter tone and the size and contour of the prostrate are noted. In female patients, vaginal examination is mandatory and should include observations on the presence or absence of vaginitis and of demonstrable stress incontinence. All patients should have a full neurological examination, including testing perianal sensation. The patient's cognitive state and mood should also be assessed.

Clinical assessment is supplemented by simple investigations including urinalysis, urine culture, glucose, tests of renal function and vaginal cytology. This initial assessment is often inadequate. Proper management may require endoscopic or urodynamic investigations.

Problems in diagnosis

The following are some of the problems encountered when attempting clinical diagnosis:

1. The symptom of stress incontinence may occur in patients with genuine stress incontinence, detrusor instability or a voiding disorder. Where due to detrusor instability there may be a delay between the stimulus of raised intra-abdominal pressure and the loss of urine. The volume of urine lost tends to be greater than in patients with genuine stress incontinence.
2. Urgency and urge incontinence are encountered not only in those with detrusor instability but also in patients with sensory urgency, genuine stress incontinence or overflow incontinence.
3. A poor urinary stream may be a consequence of outflow tract obstruction or impaired detrusor contractility. Interpretation of the urinary flow pattern requires the passage of an adequate amount of urine, usually greater than 200 ml.
4. Urinary frequency and nocturia may result from detrusor instability, sensory urgency, a high fluid intake, diabetes mellitus, diabetes insipidus, chronic renal impairment or diuretic medication. These symptoms may also occur in patients with genuine stress incontinence and voiding disorders.
5. In male patients the majority with urinary outflow tract obstruction will complain of urinary hesitancy, a poor urinary stream, post-micturition dribbling, nocturia and urgency. However, almost a third of male patients with these symptoms will have normal urodynamic findings. Nor are these symptoms significantly correlated with the degree of outflow tract obstruction. Physical findings are also unhelpful in this situation as the size of the prostrate on rectal examination does not correlate with the degree of obstruction.

Accuracy of clinical diagnosis

Studies of the accuracy of clinical diagnosis have compared the results of clinical assessment with urodynamic findings. All have found a poor correlation between the clinical and urodynamic findings. The greatest accuracy is found in women diagnosed clinically as having genuine stress incontinence. The least accuracy is usually found in women with voiding disorders.

Although the symptom of stress incontinence is 100 per cent sensitive for the diagnosis of genuine stress incontinence, it is only 65 per cent specific. In female patients with stress incontinence as their only lower urinary tract symptom, urodynamic investigations confirm the diagnosis in around 90 per cent. Studies in the elderly confirm the association in this age group. This means, however, that 10 per cent of these patients do not have genuine stress incontinence and have an underlying problem, usually detrusor instability, which is not amenable to cure by surgery for genuine stress incontinence. Unless all patients complaining of stress incontinence have prior urodynamic investigations some will undergo unnecessary and unhelpful surgery. There is controversy concerning whether or not patients with detrusor instability in addition to genuine stress incontinence should have surgery for their genuine stress incontinence. If in addition to stress incontinence a patient has urinary frequency and/or nocturia there is only a 50 per cent chance that they will prove to have genuine stress incontinence alone. Where stress incontinence and urge incontinence co-exist in the same patient the majority (80 per cent) of patients will prove to have detrusor instability. Most of the remainder have genuine stress incontinence. While some surgeons argue that it is reasonable to operate on patients with stress incontinence as their only urinary symptom, without prior urodynamic investigations, it is indefensible to proceed to surgery in patients with other lower urinary tract symptoms in addition to stress incontinence without first assessing the patient urodynamically. It must also be kept in mind that although the majority of patients with combined stress and urge incontinence have detrusor instability, a significant minority will prove to have genuine stress incontinence alone. While the management of the unstable detrusor is often unsatisfactory, surgery for genuine stress incontinence offers a higher probability of cure. To assume that all patients with combined stress and urge incontinence have unstable detrusors is to deny the minority with genuine stress incontinence a chance of a surgical cure. The lack of specificity of the symptom of stress incontinence means that urodynamic investigations are required if some patients are to avoid unnecessary surgery and others are to be offered the chance of curative surgery.

Studies have shown that the presence of a palpable bladder after micturition is highly predictive of a voiding disorder. It has also been shown that the vast majority of patients with voiding disorders do not have a palpable bladder. In one study only five out of 25 elderly females with voiding dysfunction had a palpable bladder. A palpable bladder is thus highly specific but insensitive in the identification of voiding problems. The sensitivity can be improved by measuring the residual urine. Voiding dysfunction due to outflow obstruction is rare in the female. Impaired detrusor contractility is more common. It is only in patients with complete urinary retention that a diagnosis of voiding dysfunction can be made with reasonable certainty. Urinary frequency and nocturia are the most commonly reported symptoms in female patients with disordered voiding. Other expected symptoms, such as urinary hesitancy, poor stream and a feeling of bladder fullness post-voiding are present in only a minority of female patients.

It is also known that most patients (75 per cent) with urge incontinence but no stress incontinence have detrusor instability. Most authors have concluded from this that patients with the frequency, nocturia, urgency and urge incontinence symptom complex can be assumed to have detrusor instability, providing that causes of sensory urgency have been excluded. These patients thus require endoscopic studies rather than urodynamic investigations.

Lower urinary tract symptoms are thus poor predictors of the underlying pathophysiological mechanism causing a patient's incontinence. Even when clinical findings, such as a palpable bladder or demonstrable stress incontinence, are taken into account the accuracy of clinical diagnosis remains poor. An accurate diagnosis usually requires urodynamic investigations. This is not to say, however, that prior use of these studies is a prerequisite for the management of all incontinent elderly patients.

Urodynamic investigations

The International Continence Society defines urodynamic investigations as the study of the function and dysfunction of the urinary tract by any appropriate method. It encompasses the morphological, physiological, biochemical and hydrodynamic aspects of urine transport and storage.

These studies vary in sophistication from simple pad tests to multichannel videourodynamics. Some act as screening tests, identifying those patients who require more sophisticated studies. Others provide all the information necessary for the management of the vast majority of incontinent patients. Other techniques are only available in specialist centres dealing with the more complicated cases. Some investigative techniques, while increasing our understanding of the function and dysfunction of the lower urinary tract, have not proved useful in clinical practice, and remain research tools.

Frequency volume charts

Frequency volume charts are a useful adjunct to the history. They provide a good indication of the frequency of incontinence and can give clues as to its aetiology. They also give a measure of the functional bladder capacity. The maximum voided volume on these charts shows a close correlation with the maximum cystometric capacity. The patient records when micturition occurred and the volume voided. Incontinent episodes are also noted and patients may be asked to record fluid intake. This information is collected over a 48 hour or sometimes a 7 day period.

Pad tests

Pad tests are a useful way to quantify the volume of urine lost by incontinent patients. They can be used to measure objectively the severity of a patient's incontinence. They can also be used as a research tool to measure changes in the volume of urine lost in response to therapeutic intervention. Using preweighed pads with waterproof backing the volume of urine lost in millilitres over a given period of time equates to the weight gain in grams of the pad. When used to assess the severity of incontinence the study period is usually one hour. During this time the patient carries out a series of standard manoeuvres, including drinking a half-litre of sodium-free liquid within 15 minutes, walking, climbing stairs, coughing, running on the spot for one minute, handwashing for one minute, bending and standing up from sitting. Weight gain of up to 1 g per hour may be due to sweating or vaginal discharge. Weighing errors have also to be taken into account.

A variation on the above is to change the pads every 10 minutes during the one hour period in the hope that this might give an indication as to the aetiology of the incontinence. One might expect patients with genuine stress incontinence to lose small volumes of urine into each pad. Patients with detrusor instability are expected to have infrequent losses of large volumes. Experience, however, has shown that the pattern of urine loss can be the same in both conditions. In assessing the response to intervention pad tests can be carried out over a period of days in incontinent elderly patients, the preweighed pads being changed every 2 hours. Yet another variation is the use of electronic pads. When urine is lost there is a change in the nappy's electrical capacitance which is converted electronically into a recording of urine loss in millilitres.

Post-void residual urine

This must be measured after the patient has voided with a full bladder. A high volume indicates voiding problems. An elevated post-void residual urine itself is not associated with incontinence status. Patients with vesicoureteric reflux may be incorrectly identified as having an elevated residual urine. The absence of an elevated residual urine does not exclude the presence of a voiding disorder.

Urinary flow rate

Measurement of the urinary flow rate (Fig. 7), the volume of urine voided per

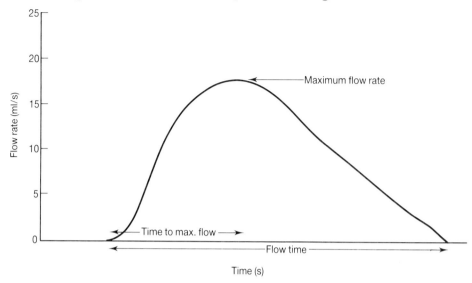

Figure 7 Urinary flow rate.

unit time which is usually expressed in millilitres per second, is a useful screening procedure which can also measure the progress of disease or its response to treatment. The patient urinates into a funnel which directs the flow on to a flowmeter. The patient usually voids in privacy to minimize any psychosomatic influences on the flow rate and pattern. The three main techniques used to measure flow rate are:

1. Electronic dip-stick method. The patient voids into a collecting chamber containing an electronic dip-stick. This has sensing electrodes which detect the change in electrical capacitance as air is replaced by urine. The change in capacitance is converted electronically into a voltage which is proportional to the volume of urine. This allows calculation of the rate at which urine is entering the chamber and thus the flow rate.
2. Gravimetric method. This is similar to the electronic dip-stick except that it is the weight of the accumulating urine which is detected and converted into an electrical signal.
3. Rotating disc method. In this technique the flow of urine is directed on to a rotating disc. On hitting the disc it tends to slow it down. The disc is kept rotating at a constant rate. The additional energy required to keep it rotating at the same rate is proportional to the urinary flow rate.

The patient must pass at least 200 ml before the urinary flow can be interpreted. Note is taken of the volume voided, the maximum flow rate, flow time, the average flow rate (voided volume divided by flow time), time to maximum flow rate and the flow pattern. The average flow rate is usually around 50 per cent of the maximum flow rate. This proportion rises in patients with outflow obstruction. The normal flow pattern is bell-shaped. Normal maximum flow rates for males are around 30–40 ml per second. For females they are of the order of 40–50 ml per second. The minimum flow rate acceptable in elderly males or females is usually around 10 ml per second. Low flow rates may not arise from outflow obstruction but from an inadequate detrusor contraction. A simple measurement of the flow rate will not distinguish these. The pattern of urinary flow may give some clues as to the underlying pathology. However, although the pattern may differ between patients with outflow obstruction and detrusor under-activity there is considerable overlap between patients. The distinction between outflow obstruction and impaired detrusor contraction usually requires simultaneous measurement of detrusor pressure and urinary flow rate. If radiographic studies are carried out at the same time the anatomical site of any obstruction can be determined. A normal flow rate does not exclude outflow obstruction as the detrusor may compensate for the obstruction. Nomograms have been constructed relating maximum flow to age, sex and the volume voided. As already mentioned, flow rates are difficult to interpret in those who persistently pass urine volumes of less than 200 ml.

Measurement of the urinary flow rate alone is sufficient for diagnosis in about half of all male patients who have uncomplicated prostatic outflow obstruction. Elderly men with symptoms suggestive of outflow obstruction who have an impaired flow rate, despite the passage of an adequate volume of urine, can be assumed to have outflow obstruction.

A significant minority of patients cannot void in situations where they have inadequate privacy. Every effort needs to be made to ensure that patients have the opportunity to void in conditions of maximum privacy.

Intravenous urogram

This has no place in the assessment of incontinent patients unless other symptoms such as haematuria are present.

Pressure measurements

In the following discussion reference will be made to pressure measurements in the bladder, the urethra and the rectum. The last is used as a measure of intra-abdominal pressure. The zero reference point for these measurements is the superior margin of the pubic symphysis. By convention the pressure is measured in centimetres of water. These pressures may be measured directly using catheter-mounted pressure transducers. More commonly the pressure is transmitted to an externally mounted pressure transducer via a fluid-filled catheter. Transducers convert mechanical parameters into an electrical signal. A pressure transducer generates an electrical signal in response to an applied pressure, the magnitude of the signal being proportional to the magnitude of the pressure.

Urethral pressure profile

Measurement of pressure along the urethra gives rise to the urethral pressure profile (Fig. 8). This is usually bell-shaped in the female, reflecting the action

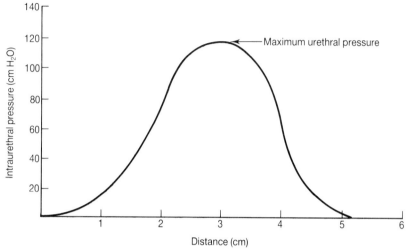

Figure 8 Urethral pressure profile.

of the rhabdosphincter. In females the urethral pressure profile falls with age. It is also lower in patients with genuine stress incontinence. There is a large overlap between normals and those with genuine stress incontinence. Because of this the urethral pressure profile is not normally an integral part of the routine assessment of incontinent patients. Its main use is as a research tool.

Cystometry

Filling cystometry (Fig. 9) measures the pressure–volume relationship of the bladder. Intravesical pressure is recorded during bladder filling. The bladder may be filled with carbon dioxide or a liquid. The latter may be water, normal saline or a radiographic contrast medium, depending on the study. Liquid has the advantages that it is physiological, can be combined with radiographic studies and can be used to test for stress incontinence. Carbon dioxide has the advantages of being quick, clean and simple. It is, however, unphysiological, irritant to the hypersensitive bladder and cannot be used to test for stress incontinence or to study pressure flow relationships. For these reasons a liquid medium is preferred.

The rate of bladder filling may be slow (less than 10 ml per minute), medium (10–100 ml per minute) or rapid (greater than 100 ml per minute). Physiological bladder filling occurs at a rate of 1 ml per minute. Most bladders are very compliant, the pressure rise being less than 15 cm of water, even at full capacity. The diagnosis of low compliance can only be made if the bladder

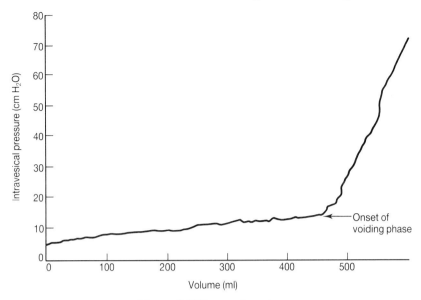

Figure 9 Filling cystometry.

is filled slowly. If it is suspected, the bladder should be filled at a rate of 10 ml per minute.

A double-lumen catheter is inserted into the patient's bladder. The post-void residual volume can be measured at this time. The bladder is filled through one channel. The pressure within the bladder is transmitted via the liquid in the second channel to an externally mounted pressure transducer. This records the pressure within the lumen of the bladder. This is a combination of the intra-abdominal pressure plus the pressure due to the detrusor. The pressure exerted via the detrusor may be active or passive. A second liquid-filled open-ended catheter is inserted into the rectum. This is covered by a protective rubber membrane to protect it from blockage by faecal material. It is connected to an external pressure transducer and measures intra-abdominal pressure. By electronically subtracting this from the intravesical pressure the detrusor pressure is obtained. This avoids the problem of artefacts due to transmitted intra-abdominal pressures if in-travesical pressure alone is measured as a representation of detrusor function.

Filling cystometry provides information on bladder compliance, bladder sensation, bladder capacity and detrusor control. Bladder capacity as mea-sured by cystometry is usually around 60 per cent of the physiological bladder capacity. Detrusor instability is indicated by pressure rises. If these are transient, they can be assumed to indicate a detrusor contraction. If the pressure rise is sustained it may be due to a sustained contraction or low compliance. Provocation of the detrusor by rapid filling, changing position or coughing does not normally lead to an unstable contraction. It may, however, provoke a detrusor contraction in a patient with detrusor instability or detrusor hyperreflexia. The incidence of detrusor instability revealed by provocation is twice that revealed by supine filling cystometry alone in young patients. In the elderly, detrusor instability is identified by supine cystometry alone in 90 per cent of cases.

The first sensation of bladder filling normally occurs at around 150 ml, the urge to void usually occurs around 350 ml, and bladder capacity is usually between 400 and 500 ml.

Pressure flow studies

After filling cystometry, micturition can be studied. The filling catheter is removed from the bladder but the catheter connected to the pressure transducer remains. With allowance being made for the presence of this tube in the urethra the flow rate is measured. At the same time the intravesical pressure is recorded. This allows distinction between low flow rates due to impaired contractility and low flow rates due to outflow obstruction. Thus a low flow rate combined with high detrusor pressure suggests outflow obstruction. A low flow rate combined with a low detrusor pressure suggests an under-active detrusor. Before the bladder is empty the patient can also be tested to see if the symptom and sign of stress incontinence is due to genuine stress incontinence or to detrusor instability. The patient is asked to cough in the supine and then erect position with a full bladder. If leakage of urine occurs without a rise in detrusor pressure, genuine stress incontinence is diagnosed. In males the maximum detrusor pressure during micturition is normally 30–40 cm of water. The normal female voids at a lower pressure because outflow resistance is lower.

Videocystourethrography (VCU)

Further sophistication is added by combining filling cystometry, tests for stress incontinence and pressure flow studies with fluoroscopic screening. In this case a contrast medium is used instead of sterile water or normal saline. This technique allows the additional identification of bladder trabeculation, vesicoureteric reflux and bladder diverticuli. If outflow obstruction is present the anatomical site can be visualized. The study is usually done with a camera over the multichannel recorder displaying the intra-abdominal pressure, the intravesical pressure, the detrusor pressure and the flow rate. A mixing unit displays the picture from the camera on one half of a television screen and the simultaneous X-ray image on the other half. These images are recorded for later scrutiny.

While often referred to as the gold standard of urodynamic studies on incontinent patients, VCU is not necessary for the investigation of the majority of incontinent patients. Its use can be reserved for the more complex patients such as those who have already had failed surgery for incontinence, those with voiding problems and in those with neurological disease.

Procedure for a VCU

A VCU starts with the patient being asked to void into a flowmeter. The patient is then placed supine on the X-ray table and a fluid-filled catheter, protected by a fingerstall and connected to an external pressure transducer, is inserted into the rectum to record intra-abdominal pressure. A two-channel catheter is inserted into the bladder. One filled with fluid is connected to an external pressure transducer and records the intravesical pressure. The detrusor pressure is derived electronically by subtracting the intra-abdominal pressure from the intravesical pressure. The second channel is used to drain the bladder thus recording the residual volume. Contrast medium is then run in, usually at a rate of 100 ml per minute. The patient reports the first desire to void and when the desire to void is strong. Note is taken of any unstable detrusor activity. Fluoroscopic screening allows identification of diverticuli, vesicoureteric reflux and bladder trabeculation. When bladder capacity has been reached the patient is tested for stress incontinence. It can be seen if this is due to genuine stress incontinence or a provoked unstable contraction. The patient is then moved into the erect position and again asked to cough. The filling catheter in the bladder is removed and the patient is asked to void into a flowmeter while the detrusor pressure is noted.

Electromyography

Electromyography of the urethral striated muscle can be carried out using needle or surface electrodes, the former being more accurate. These studies may be helpful in some patients with neuropathic disorders of the lower urinary tract where they provide information on the external sphincter during voiding. They allow separation of functional distal obstruction due to striated muscle activity from that due to smooth muscle activity. In general these studies are rarely important in determining clinical management and EMG is used primarily as a research tool. If used during routine urodynamic studies the patient may be incorrectly diagnosed as having detrusor sphincter dyssynergia as it is normal for patients to contract the pelvic floor muscles in the presence of an unstable detrusor contraction. This mistake is less likely to be made if the operator remembers that detrusor external sphincter dys-synergia is very rare in the absence of overt neurological disease.

Ambulatory urodynamic studies

Ambulatory urodynamic studies are a recent advance, having the advantage that they record bladder activity during normal filling cylces. The hope is that this will improve the diagnostic rate. Their role in the assessment of incontinent patients is currently under investigation.

Cystoscopy

Endoscopic examination of the lower urinary tract is indicated in patients with urge incontinence but no stress incontinence in order to exclude the various causes of sensory urgency. Cystoscopy and IVP are mandatory in patients with haematuria. Once the causes of sensory urgency have been excluded, patients can be assumed to have an unstable detrusor.

Ultrasound

Ultrasound studies have been used to localize the bladder neck and measure its descent with raised intra-abdominal pressure. Ultrasound can also be used to measure the post-void residual urine.

The indications for urodynamic studies in elderly female patients

Despite the difficulties involved in making a clinical diagnosis it is not necessary to perform urodynamic investigations on all incontinent patients before initiating treatment. As already mentioned the vast majority of female patients with stress incontinence as their only lower urinary tract symptom have genuine stress incontinence. It has been argued that urodynamic studies are mandatory on these patients before surgery for genuine stress incontinence if the small number of these patients who have detrusor instability and no evidence of genuine stress incontinence are to be saved unnecessary surgery. While this is undoubtedly good practice it is not always practicable and many patients currently have surgery for genuine stress incontinence without prior urodynamic studies. If patients with stress incontinence have other lower urinary tract symptoms the incidence of diagnoses other than genuine stress incontinence becomes appreciable and such patients should undoubtedly have urodynamic studies before any surgical intervention. Patients who have had failed surgery for genuine stress incontinence should also have urodynamic investigations before being subjected to further surgery.

Patients with urge incontinence but no stress incontinence can be assumed to have detrusor instability, providing the causes of sensory urgency have been excluded. The most difficult diagnostic problem is the identification of female patients with voiding disorders. The presence of a palpable bladder after micturition is a relatively specific but insensitive way to screen for voiding disorders.

In an attempt to rationalize the use of urodynamic studies in the investigation and management of incontinent elderly women, Hilton and Stanton prepared an algorithm based on the clinical and urodynamic findings in 100 incontinent elderly women (Fig. 10). The urodynamic studies showed that 29

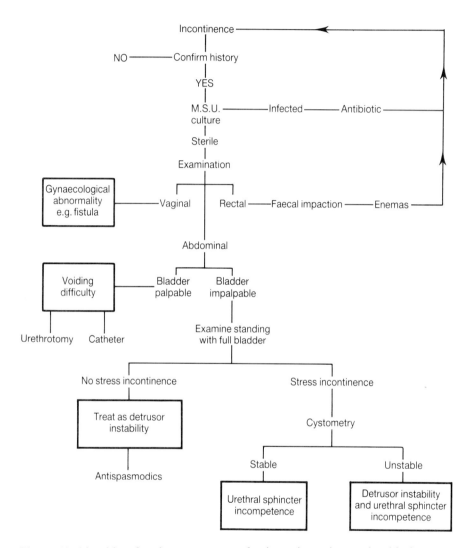

Figure 10 Algorithm for the assessment of urinary incontinence in elderly women (reproduced with permission from Hilton and Stanton, 1981).

of the patients had detrusor instability alone, 30 had genuine stress incontinence alone, 10 had detrusor instability and genuine stress incontinence, 14 had voiding problems and 4 had no detectable abnormality; 3 proved impossible to assess. Ten had a palpable bladder with a post-void residual urine in excess of 300 ml. Based on their findings they prepared an algorithm, the main features of which were: (a) patients with a palpable bladder were assumed to have a voiding disorder and were not subjected to urodynamic studies; (b) patients with stress incontinence had urodynamic studies; (c) patients without stress incontinence or a palpable bladder were assumed to have detrusor instability. The algorithm was then applied retrospectively to the 100 incontinent women. From a diagnostic point of view the algorithm gave an accuracy of 83 per cent. The correct treatment would have been initiated in 95 per cent. Urodynamic studies would have been required in only 40 per cent of patients. Eastwood and Warrell assessed the validity of this approach in a prospective study of 65 elderly incontinent women. They used the algorithm to make a clinical diagnosis. In doing this they introduced one modification. Patients with stress incontinence as their only lower urinary tract symptom were assumed to have genuine stress incontinence. They then performed urodynamic studies to assess the accuracy of the algorithm. Had they used the algorithm as originally proposed, they would have made the correct diagnosis in 89 per cent of cases and management would have been correct in 95 per cent. Urodynamic studies would only have been required in 18 per cent of the patients. In both of these studies a significant minority of patients with voiding problems would have been undiagnosed. This was the only important drawback.

Urodynamic studies are thus indicated in:

1. female patients with stress incontinence and any other lower urinary tract symptom—if practical they should be performed on all those with stress incontinence before surgery;
2. patients who have had failed surgery for genuine stress incontinence;
3. patients with voiding difficulties;
4. patients with neuropathic bladder disorders;
5. some specialists recommend urodynamic studies for patients with presumed detrusor instability who fail to respond satisfactorily to treatment.

Obviously these guidelines do not apply to those whose mental or physical frailty makes them unsuitable for operative intervention. As with all good medical practice invasive investigation should only be carried out when the result is likely to affect management. It would be unreasonable to inflict full urodynamic studies on a cognitively impaired 85-year-old female patient with mixed stress and urge incontinence. There is no point in trying to demonstrate that these symptoms are due to genuine stress incontinence if surgery for this condition is out of the question. It is much more reasonable to assume that she has detrusor instability and manage her accordingly. These studies are not without complications. The X-ray exposure is similar to that of an IVP if VCU is performed. The main risk is infection. Cystometry has been shown to lead to urinary tract infection in over 20 per cent of elderly patients. In addition, the procedure may be uncomfortable for the patient. Urodynamic studies on elderly patients are often time-consuming and expensive of medical nursing and radiographic time. Their use is justified only if the patient is likely to benefit from the result.

The indications for urodynamic studies in elderly male patients

In the assessment of incontinent male patients urodynamic investigations may be of help in a number of situations, as outlined below.

Stress incontinence in the male is rare and is usually the result of neurological damage or surgical trauma. Its assessment usually warrants urodynamic studies.

As already discussed, history and clinical examination by themselves cannot be relied upon for the diagnosis of prostatic outflow obstruction. A poor urinary stream may result from detrusor instability alone if the patient persistently passes small volumes of urine. Nor is the size of the prostate on rectal examination helpful. An enlarged prostate may be associated with no obstruction while a normal-sized prostate on rectal examination may co-exist with marked outflow obstruction. Cystourethroscopy may also be misleading. If outflow obstruction is due to a dyssynergic bladder neck the endoscopic appearances may be normal. Bladder neck dyssynergia is a dysfunctional disorder which occurs in a younger age group than prostatic hypertrophy. The bladder neck paradoxically tightens as the detrusor contracts. It is sometimes difficult to know if early lateral lobe encroachment on the urethra is producing a functional obstruction. Although endoscopy cannot always prove or exclude bladder outflow obstruction, it is essential to identify the cause of any obstruction.

Because of these problems it is mandatory to at least check the flow rate on all patients being considered for prostatic resection, the only exception to this being a patient in retention.

Studies have shown that, where male patients are being assessed for outflow tract obstruction, an IVP, endoscopy and, if indicated, prostatic biopsy will lead to the correct diagnosis in over 90 per cent of patients. Resort to VCU is required on only a small minority of cases. These patients, who tend to be in the younger age group, are usually found to have bladder neck dyssynergia or else are shown to have no evidence of outflow tract obstruction.

In male patients with outflow tract obstruction the symptoms of frequency, nocturia and urgency are not directly due to the outflow obstruction except in the occasional patient with a large residual urine associated with borderline retention. These irritative symptoms may result from associated hypersensitive conditions such as bladder calculi or infection but they are usually due to associated detrusor instability. Over half of all patients with significant outflow tract obstruction will have detrusor instability. It has been suggested that there is little point in identifying which patients with outflow tract obstruction are also unstable as this will not influence management. However, it is important to show objectively that male patients with a mixture of 'obstructive' and 'irritative' symptoms are indeed obstructed, as such patients may have detrusor instability alone. In the older male patient it is in the identification of those with non-obstructive detrusor instability that voiding studies are of particular value. Unfortunately, in very elderly males being assessed urodynamically for obstruction these investigations are often inconclusive because of difficulties in getting the patient to void under test conditions, and because the volumes voided may be too small to allow adequate interpretation.

A major problem in patients with outflow obstruction and bladder instability is the identification of those likely to benefit from operative intervention, as persistent detrusor instability is the most common cause of post-prostatecomy incontinence. This distinction cannot be made by the routine urodynamic investigations already described. A number of tests have been reported as being useful in predicting those patients whose incontinence is likely to benefit from operation. A prolonged evoked response to electrical stimulation of the posterior urethra or the persistence of detrusor instability after insertion of intravesical lignocaine have both been reported as good predictors of failed surgery as far as the detrusor instability is concerned. Relief of the outflow obstruction, however, remains a desirable end of itself. Because of the reduced resistance and improved flow, urine loss may be more marked post-operatively.

Male patients with an under-active detrusor may complain of symptoms suggestive of outflow obstruction. Patients with a large residual urine may be diagnosed as having an under-active detrusor if there is no obvious obstruction on endoscopic examination. In this situation urodynamic studies may be an additional aid to management. While some of these patients will be shown to have an under-active detrusor with normal outflow resistance, in others the outflow resistance may be unexpectedly high and associated with a partially decompensated detrusor. Obstructive detrusor decompensation often recovers following relief of the obstruction.

A problem also encountered by physicians in geriatric medicine is the patient with incontinence due to detrusor instability who has a neurological lesion in addition to outflow tract obstruction. There is no way of distinguishing with certainty if the instability is secondary to the obstruction or the neurological lesion. If outflow obstruction is confirmed and operated upon, just over half of these patients will be less incontinent post-operatively.

From the above it can be seen that, apart from measurement of the flow rate and residual urine, urodynamic investigations have only a small part to play in the management of incontinent elderly males. They are required in the few with stress incontinence and in those with symptoms of outflow obstruction in whom endoscopy fails to reveal any obstructive lesion. In this case their value is to demonstrate the presence of unobstructed detrusor instability. They are also indicated in some patients with neurological lesions, for example, those with traumatic spinal cord damage and multiple sclerosis. As with elderly female patients the decision to proceed to invasive urodynamic studies is only justified if the result is likely to affect management.

References

Bates CP, Corney E. Synchronous cine pressure flow cystography: a method of routine urodynamic investigation. *Br. J. Radiol.* 1971; **44:** 44–50.

Drutz HB, Mandell F. Urodynamic analysis of urinary incontinence symptoms in women. *Gynaecology* 1979; **134:** 789–792.

Eastwood HDH, Warrell R. Urinary incontinence in the elderly female: prediction in diagnosis and outcome of management. *Age Ageing* 1984; **13:** 230–234.

Farrar DJ, Whiteside DG, Osborne JL, Turner-Warwick A. Urodynamic analysis of micturition symptoms in the female. *Surg. Gynaecol. Obstet.* 1975; **141:** 875–881.

Herbison AE, Farundorfur MR, Walton, JK. Association between symptomatology and uroflometry in benign prostatic hypertrophy. *Br. J. Urol.* 1988; **62:** 427–430.

Hilton P. Stanton SL. Algorithmic method for assessing urinary incontinence in elderly women. *Br. Med. J.* 1981; **282:** 940–942.

Jarvis GJ, Hall S, Stamp S, Millar DR, Johnson A. An assessment of urodynamic examination in incontinent women. *Br. J. Obstet. Gynaecol.* 1980; **87:** 893–896.

Kong TK, Morris JA, Robinson JM, Brocklehurst JC. Predicting urodynamic dysfunction from clinical features in incontinent elderly women. *Age Ageing* 1990; **19:** 257–263.

McGuire EJ, Lytton B, Kohoran EI, Pepe V. The value of urodynamic testing in stress urinary incontinence. *J. Urol.* 1980; **124:** 256–258.

Chapter 5 _____

Voiding regimes

Various voiding regimes have been introduced for the management of detrusor instability and hyperreflexia. Some are curative, some palliative and others of purely academic interest. All have the advantage of being safe. Most incontinent elderly patients who are institutionalized, be it in a residential home, nursing home or in a hospital, are on a voiding regime. This is invariably initiated as a matter of routine by the care assistants or nursing staff without any prior input from the medical profession. It is often the only treatment that the patient is receiving for incontinence. This chapter reviews the theories behind these regimes, their efficacy and their place in the management of incontinence.

Timed voiding

Regular timed voiding is the mainstay of the management of the incontinent elderly in residential care, nursing homes and hospitals. It involves the nursing staff taking patients to the toilet at regular intervals, usually two-hourly, throughout the day. Patients may also be toileted during the night. Most patients will not tolerate being woken more than twice during the night. The purpose of toileting patients with detrusor instability or detrusor hyperreflexia is to have them empty their bladder before the onset of an involuntary contraction. Patients with detrusor instability get the urge to void at the onset of the unstable contraction. This usually leaves them with an inadequate amount of time in which to reach and use the toilet. By having the patient empty his or her bladder before the volume at which unstable contractions are precipitated is reached it is hoped to maintain continence.

It is important that patients are toileted at the appointed time, even if they have lost urine within the preceding hour. This may have been an unstable contraction. These unstable contractions often fail to empty the bladder and a substantial volume of urine may remain in it. Unless the patient empties her bladder, the volume at which an unstable contraction occurs will be reached before the patient is due to be toileted again. Timed voiding will fail if patients have unstable contractions at a low level of bladder filling as they will be incontinent before being toileted. It may also fail if the patient is unable to void voluntarily or has stress-induced unstable contractions. The act of standing her to take her to the toilet may itself precipitate incontinence.

The efficacy of timed voiding and the factors which influence the outcome have not been adequately studied. This is surprising when one considers the tremendous amount of nursing time and effort expended on the process. In one trial the authors studied its efficacy in 58 incontinent continuing-care male patients. Unfortunately, not all of the patients had detrusor instability, less than half completed the study and the magnitude of the improvement was not reported. Other studies have had small numbers or have combined timed voiding with drug therapy. This makes it impossible to know the contribution, if any, that the voiding regime made to the patient's improvement.

In residential homes staff tend to toilet residents before and after meals, as they go to and from the dining room. As there are normally limited toilet facilities adjacent to the dining room, this invariably leads to the undignified spectacle of long queues of residents being herded to and from the toilet by the care staff. No-one has objectively studied the impact of this practice on the level of continence among residents. It is obviously time-consuming for the care staff. Most believe it to be worthwhile and to have significantly reduced the level of incontinence in the home. They often cite the loss of an all-prevailing smell of stale urine in the home in support of this.

Nursing staff who deal regularly with frail, physically disabled elderly patients will automatically toilet those they identify as having troublesome incontinence. On the other hand, ambulant sensible incontinent patients who look after their own personal hygiene and change their clothes if wet are rarely toileted.

Although its efficacy has not been adequately assessed, regular timed and voiding appears to be the easiest regime to use in an institutional setting, particularly when dealing with a population with a high prevalence of cognitive impairment and physical disability. With timed voiding no attempt is made to alter bladder function. Its purpose is to minimize the effects of detrusor instability, not to cure it.

Habit retraining

Habit retraining is a variation on the timed voiding regime. It involves assessing whether or not the patient is wet or dry at certain specified times and whether or not urine is then voided. If the patient is found to have been incontinent, observations are adjusted to an earlier time to ensure continence. If the patient is found to be continent and does not pass urine, that time on the schedule is omitted. The aim is to prepare an individualized toileting regime. It is time-consuming and only possible where there is a high staff–patient ratio. It is unlikely to find favour on most wards and in most nursing or residential homes. In one study of habit retraining only a third of the patients improved. In another study of 40 patients in a continuing-care institution, habit retraining combined with behaviour therapy had no impact on the level of incontinence. It should be noted that the term habit retraining is used by some authors as a synonym for bladder drill.

Prompted voiding and behaviour therapy

Here the patient is prompted to use the toilet but is not taken to the toilet unless she takes the hint and requests to be toileted. Social approval and/or material reward is delivered if the patient is dry or responds to the prompt and requests to be toileted. Social disapproval is delivered or social approval and material rewards withheld where the patient is found to have been incontinent or fails to respond to the prompt. The aim of this approach is to modify the patient's toileting behaviour. Most successful studies have involved psychotic patients and the mentally handicapped. Where social and material reinforcement has been used in an attempt to lessen incontinence among the elderly with dementia, the results have been disappointing. This is not surprising as their memory deficit is likely to make any attempt at reinforcement futile. Even where success has been claimed it has usually taken over six weeks of behaviour therapy to attain and the reduction in the number of incontinent episodes has been of the order of 25 per cent. This seems a small return for the effort required.

Bladder drill

Bladder drill is a psychomedical treatment based on the assumption that the idiopathic unstable bladder is a functional disorder. Unlike timed voiding where the aim is to minimize the effect of unstable detrusor activity, the purpose here is to teach the patient to regain control over her bladder. She is instructed to pass urine at specified times, usually starting with one- or two-hourly intervals. She ignores sensations from her bladder and waits until the interval is up before voiding. She cannot go earlier. She either resists the urge to void or is incontinent. Various distracting techniques can be used by patients to assist in resisting the urge to void. These include pelvic floor contractions, controlled breathing exercises and mathematical problem solving. Patients are encouraged to wear normal clothes and to avoid using protective garments in order to stimulate them to try harder. The patients then void at the scheduled time whether or not they have the urge to void. When a patient can successfully defer voiding for the specified period of time, the interval is increased by 30 minutes. This is continued until she can maintain continence for 4 hours. No instructions are given concerning nocturnal voiding. The use of bladder drill in the management of incontinence due to idiopathic detrusor instability was popularized by Frewen.

When it was first introduced the patients were admitted to hospital. It is now used as an out-patient procedure. It is not indicated for those with detrusor hyperreflexia.

There have been many trials on the use of bladder drill in female patients with idiopathic detrusor instability. Most have reported cure rates of 60–80 per cent at 3 months. Despite good short-term results, 10–15 per cent of patients relapse in the long-term. Relapse rates are even higher in the elderly. Cure is usually associated with resolution of urodynamic abnormalities. Where patients with organic brain disease have been included they have failed to respond. Although many trials have included patients over 70 years of age, most have failed to study the effects of age on outcome. There have been few studies looking specifically at older women. In one such study the authors reported a cure rate of 46 per cent. Unfortunately, all of the patients received imipramine and it is not possible to separate the benefit resulting from the bladder drill from that due to the drug. In a later study by the same authors, bladder drill plus imipramine was compared with bladder drill plus placebo. There was no statistically significant difference between the two groups. Twenty of the 34 patients regained continence. Other smaller studies without concomitant drug therapy have shown bladder drill to be useful in older women with detrusor instability.

Bladder drill has also been used to treat urge incontinence in patients with primary vesical sensory urgency. These patients with frequency, nocturia, urgency and urge incontinence have stable bladders on urodynamic testing and no evidence of any pathology on endoscopic examination. The aetiology of this condition is unknown. Bladder drill appears to be as effective in these patients as it is in those with unstable detrusors. The high response rate of primary vesical sensory urgency to bladder drill indicates that it, too, is probably a psychosomatic problem.

The use of bladder drill in male patients with idiopathic detrusor instability has not been adequately assessed. Bladder drill appears to be a useful and safe treatment for female patients with idiopathic detrusor instability. Symptomatic cure is usually associated with a reversion of urodynamic abnormalities to normal.

Biofeedback

Biofeedback is a form of learning in which a patient is placed in a closed feedback loop in which a normally unconscious physiological process is made available to them as a visual or auditory stimulus. It has been used in the treatment of idiopathic detrusor instability. The detrusor pressure is measured by means of cystometry and converted into visual and auditory stimuli. The patient learns voluntary control by observing the effects of attempts to control bladder pressure changes. They learn to inhibit voluntarily unstable detrusor contractions. Restoration of continence is usually associated with reversion of urodynamic abnormalities to normal. Biofeedback does not work in patients with severe detrusor instability. Cure rates are similar to those of bladder drill. It has been used with some success in elderly patients but is very time-consuming and requires highly motivated and intelligent patients. It offers no advantages over the much simpler bladder drill.

Biofeedback can also be used to try to improve the results of physiotherapy in the management of genuine stress incontinence. Physiotherapy in this situation is aimed at trying to get the patient to contract her periurethral muscles selectively while inhibiting contraction of the abdominal muscles. Biofeedback is provided by using a perineometer (a balloon inserted into the vagina which is connected to an external pressure gauge). It records the strength of pelvic floor muscle contraction. Trials have produced conflicting results on the benefits of using a perineometer.

Hypnotherapy

Hypnosis has also been used in the treatment of idiopathic detrusor instability. As with biofeedback and bladder drill, restoration of continence is usually associated with reversion of cystometric abnormalities to normal. Cure rates are similar to those of bladder drill over which it seems to have no particular advantage.

The success of bladder drill, biofeedback and hypnosis in the management of idiopathic detrusor instability lends support to the hypothesis that psychological factors are important in its causation.

Conclusion

Regular timed voiding is the voiding regime of choice for patients with detrusor hyperreflexia. Where incontinence persists because patients are already wet when nursing staff come to toilet them, drug therapy can be added. The aim of this is to try to defer the onset of unstable contractions long enough to allow successful toileting. Regular toileting is a safe therapeutic regime, easy to introduce in an institutional setting, which reduces the overall level of incontinence and may spare some patients any incontinent episodes.

For patients with idiopathic detrusor instability, bladder drill is the therapy of choice. This includes those elderly patients with over-active bladders who have no evidence of neurological disease. The additional benefits, if any, of biofeedback, hypnotherapy, behaviour therapy and bladder retraining are not worth the extra effort.

References

Cardozo LD, Abrams PD, Stanton SL, Feneley RCL. Idiopathic bladder instability treated by biofeedback. *Br. J. Urol.* 1978; **50:** 521–523.

Castelden CM, Duffin HM. Guidelines for controlling urinary incontinence without drugs or catheters. *Age Ageing* 1981; **10:** 186–190.

Castelden CM, Duffin HM, Golati RS. Double-blind study of imipramine and placebo for incontinence due to bladder instability. *Age Ageing* 1986; **15:** 299–303.

Freeman RM, Baxby K. Hypnotherapy for incontinence caused by the unstable detrusor. *Br. Med. J.* 1982; **284:** 1831–1834.

Frewen WK. An objective assessment of the unstable bladder of psychosomatic origin. *Br. J. Urol.* 1978; **50:** 246–249.

Hardy VM, Capuano EF, Worsam BD. The effect of care programmes on the dependency status of elderly residents in an extended care setting. *J. Adv. Nurs.* 1982; **7:** 295–306.

Holmes DM, Stone AR, Barry BR, Richards LJ, Stevenson TP. Bladder training three years on. *Br. J. Urol.* 1983; **55:** 660–664.

Jarvis GJ. The management of urinary incontinence due to primary vesical sensory urgency by bladder drill. *Br. J. Urol.* 1982; **54:** 374–376.

Sogbein SK, Awad SA. Behavioural treatment of urinary incontinence in geriatric patients. *Can. Med. Assoc. J.* 1982; **127:** 863–864.

Tarrier N, Larner S. The effects of manipulation of social reinforcement on toilet requests on a geriatric ward. *Age Ageing* 1983; **12:** 234–239.

Chapter 6

The drug treatment of urinary incontinence

Drugs are available for the treatment of urinary incontinence due to detrusor instability, detrusor hyperreflexia, genuine stress incontinence and the under-active detrusor (Table 2). Despite the rationale behind the introduction of many of the drugs and the large literature on their use, it remains difficult to obtain a balanced view of their efficacy and thus of their place in the management of incontinent elderly patients. Most of this difficulty arises because of the poor calibre of many of the published drug trials.

When assessing the efficacy of a drug in the management of lower urinary tract dysfunction it is necessary to ensure that the patients have been accurately diagnosed. It is also important to measure change objectively rather than relying solely on the patient's subjective response. The use of urodynamic studies to diagnose accurately the problem and as an objective measure of the effect of the drug being tested on the relevant lower urinary tract function is thus mandatory. In many of the early drug trials, urodynamic investigations were not used. Even where they were used to make an accurate diagnosis some early investigators failed to use them to measure outcome, preferring instead to rely on the patient's subjective response. Where change has been measured urodynamically it has not always been subjected to statistical analysis.

In many of the trials on the use of drugs in the management of the over-active detrusor most, if not all, of the patients have had idiopathic detrusor instability. This is a condition with a very high placebo response. In trials, the placebo response has varied from 40 to 80 per cent. Unless the drug has been subjected to a properly designed double-blind placebo-controlled trial no conclusions can be drawn concerning its efficacy.

Much of the published work suffers from other basic flaws in design or analysis. Numbers have often been very small. Small trials require large observed differences to be statistically significant. In addition, small trials with non-significant differences are less likely to be accepted for publication than small trials with significant differences, which can lead to publication bias. Some authors have reported that patients were symptomatically improved or that there was an improvement in urodynamic parameters without defining what was considered to constitute an improvement. In other reports, no attempt has been made to subject the data to statistical analysis. Few studies have checked on patients' compliance and in fewer still have the authors attempted dose ranging. Most drug trials to date have been short-term and the longer term benefit, if any, of many of the drugs has yet to be established.

A distinction has to be made between statistical significance and clinical significance. It may be possible to demonstrate that a drug leads to a statistically significant increase in the volume at which involuntary contractions occur. This improvement may not be of much benefit to the patient if it results in her being incontinent five instead of six times a day. It may, however, be helpful if the patient is also on a regular timed voiding regime which is failing because the patient has already been incontinent by the time the nursing staff come to toilet her; the addition of the drug may defer voiding long enough to allow toileting to be successful.

Drugs and the unstable detrusor

Many of the drugs introduced for the management of detrusor instability and detrusor hyperreflexia have more than one possible beneficial mode of action. This has the advantage of maximizing benefit while minimizing potential side-effects. In general, they act on the efferent parasympathetic supply to the detrusor or on the muscle itself. Anticholinergic agents, direct smooth muscle relaxants, calcium antagonists, prostaglandin inhibitors and agents with combined effects are available. The anticholinergic agents used have mainly antimuscarinic effects. Their use is based on the fact that the main physiological stimulus for detrusor contraction is stimulation of post-ganglionic parasympathetic cholinergic receptors on the detrusor smooth muscle cells. Smooth muscle relaxants act directly on these cells at a site distal to the cholinergic receptors. Calcium antagonists act by inhibiting calcium influx into smooth muscle cells and by inhibiting the mobilization of calcium from intracellular stores. Contractile protein activation depends on an increased concentration of cytoplasmic calcium. By inhibiting its availability these drugs inhibit muscle contractility.

In using these drugs it may prove impossible to obtain a worthwhile effect on the bladder without significant side-effects. The commonest side-effects are anticholinergic, e.g., dry mouth, blurred vision, confusion, or constipation.

The efficacy of drugs in the management of detrusor instability and detrusor hyperreflexia is usually assessed by:

(a) subjective measures in which patient preferences are recorded using rating or visual analogue scales;

(b) micturition charts on which the patient records the frequency of voluntary micturition and the number of incontinent epidodes;

(c) urodynamic studies paying particular attention to the volume at first urge to micturate, maximum bladder capacity and residual urine.

It is fair to say that while patients may improve on these drugs they seldom by themselves lead to continence. They may succeed in increasing the volume at which unstable contractions occur and they may decrease the amplitude of involuntary contractions but they rarely restore stability. Although often used alone, their overall effect on the incontinent elderly is minor and they should be used in combination with a suitable voiding regime.

Oxybutynin hydrochloride

Oxybutynin hydrochloride has been used for the management of detrusor instability and detrusor hyperreflexia for over 15 years in the USA. Until 1991 it was only available on a named patient basis in the UK. Its present very small share of the market in the UK is likely to change with the recent withdrawal of its main competitor terodiline. Oxybutynin hydrochloride has combined anticholinergic and smooth muscle relaxant properties. It also acts as a local anaesthetic. The contribution, if any, of this to its effects on the unstable detrusor is unknown. It is rapidly absorbed when given orally. It is also rapidly eliminated, having a short half-life which is slightly prolonged in the elderly. Although the usual recommended dosage is 5 mg three times a day, a dose of 5 mg twice daily suffices in the elderly. This relatively safe drug is rapidly metabolized in the liver, its main metabolite having comparable anticholinergic properties. The majority of patients experience side-effects which are usually anticholinergic and cease on stopping the drug. Around a quarter of patients stop taking the drug because they find the side-effects, particularly the dry mouth, intolerable.

There have been many studies of its efficacy in the management of detrusor instability and hyperreflexia. Some of these have been seriously flawed in design or interpretation but the better studies have shown a significant improvement in symptoms and urodynamic parameters. The drug is significantly better than placebo at reducing the frequency of micturition, reducing incontinence episodes, increasing the volume at first desire to void and increasing bladder capacity. Its efficacy in the elderly has not been adequately assessed. Results from the few patients studied to date have been unimpressive.

The intravesical administration of oxybutynin has been used successfully in the management of patients with neuropathic bladder disorders who empty their bladders by clean intermittent self-catheterization and who remain incontinent because of persisting detrusor hyperreflexia. When given by this route there is a marked reduction in the incidence of anticholinergic side-effects.

Terodiline

At the time of writing (1992), terodiline is the most widely prescribed drug for the management of incontinence in the UK, where it is taken by over 70 000 patients. Around 2 million patients use it world-wide. It is, however, being 'withdrawn' by its manufacturers because of concerns raised by the Committee of Safety on Medicines. Through its yellow card scheme the Committee identified 17 patients on terodiline who had episodes of ventricular tachycardia, mainly of the 'Torsades de Pointes' variety. There were a further three reports of heart block and four of bradycardia. Three patients had cardiac arrests and five required pacing. The risk of arrhythmias was associated with age greater than 75 years, ischaemic heart disease, hypokalaemia and the co-prescription of diuretics, tricyclic antidepressants and anti-psychotic medication. In none of the original reports did the arrhythmia prove fatal. Subsequent reports did, however, include fatalities and this led the Company to announce its withdrawal of the drug.

Terodiline was originally introduced as an anti-anginal agent. It has anticholinergic and calcium antagonist properties, both demonstrable within roughly the same concentration range. The recommended dosage was 25 mg twice daily but therapeutic serum levels could be obtained in the elderly using half this dose. The mean half-life of the drug in the frail elderly is 190 hours.

Terodiline is the most researched drug introduced for the management of incontinence. In most studies significant symptomatic improvement was found when the drug was compared to placebo. Patients have reported a reduction in the frequency of micturition and in the number of incontinence episodes. These symptomatic improvements have not always been matched by corresponding improvements in urodynamic parameters. The trend towards improvement in bladder capacity and bladder volume at first desire to void has in general been more marked in the patients receiving terodiline than in those on placebo. It has been suggested that the disparity between the subjective and objective findings may be due to the unphysiological rate of bladder filling used when performing urodynamic studies. Ambulatory studies with the bladder filling at a normal rate would be required to resolve this. In what will probably prove to be the last trial of the drug in the incontinent elderly it was found to be no better than placebo. Although the number of patients was relatively small the authors were able to conclude that its effects, if any, in this age group were small. Considering the doubts that exist regarding its efficacy in the incontinent elderly and the seriousness of the reported side-effects to which the elderly are particularly susceptible, its use in this age group cannot be recommended should it ever be re-marketed.

Emepromium bromide

Emepromium bromide is an anticholinergic agent whose popularity in the management of detrusor instability rested on favourable reports from poorly designed and analysed drug trials. In recent well-designed studies, researchers were unable to demonstrate any objective benefit from the drug. This may have been because it is so poorly absorbed when given orally. High doses given parenterally were shown to be effective but the effects were too short-lasting to be of clinical value. The drug is no longer available.

Flavoxate

Flavoxate is a smooth muscle relaxant whose popularity, like that of emepromium bromide, rested on favourable reports from poorly designed and analysed trials. As with emepromium bromide, it is the better designed and analysed trials which have produced the evidence against it being effective.

Propantheline

Propantheline is a synthetic analogue of atropine with antimuscarinic and antinicotinic effects. Experimental studies in animals and studies using parenteral propantheline in humans have shown it to have an effect on the unstable detrusor. There is a relative paucity of clinical data on the use of the oral agent. It is poorly and unreliably absorbed from the gastrointestinal tract. In one study the dose was increased until side-effects developed or until it was effective. Half of the patients developed urinary retention. Around a third of the patients were cured by propantheline alone, one-third required the addition of intermittent catheterization and one-third required permanent catheterization. Its efficacy has been compared with that of oxybutynin in a number of studies. These have found oxybutynin to be the more effective drug. One large study, in which propantheline appeared to be no better than placebo, has been criticized because of the relatively low dose of propantheline prescribed. It is usually started in a dose of 15 mg four times a day, increasing to 30 mg four times a day.

Imipramine

Imipramine has a variety of actions which may be of benefit in patients with detrusor instability. It has peripheral antimuscarinic effects. It also has sympathomimetic effects. As a beta stimulant it leads to detrusor relaxation and as an alpha stimulator it may increase bladder outflow resistance. It is also said to have a central action, to have direct smooth muscle relaxing effects, and to have calcium antagonist activity. Animal experiments suggest that parenteral imipramine reduces detrusor contractility but human studies failed to show a significant effect on urodynamic parameters; this difference may be due to species differences. Early studies reporting beneficial results from oral imipramine contained very small numbers of patients in addition to other more fundamental flaws in design. More recently Castelden and co-workers have reported the outcome of treating 95 elderly patients with imipramine. Nearly half of the patients regained continence. However, the patients had bladder drill in addition to the drug and it is impossible to separate the effects of the drug from those of the toileting regime. Nor was a placebo used as this was not a prospective drug trial but was a report of their experiences in a geriatric incontinence clinic. In a later study the same authors performed a double-blind placebo-controlled trial comparing imipramine with placebo. Both groups had bladder drill in addition to their drug therapy. There was no stastically significant difference between the two groups, although more of the patients on imipramine regained continence. The case in favour of using this drug remains unproven despite its widespread use. Its use may be associated with troublesome side-effects, including postural hypotension, dry mouth, constipation, confusion and sedation.

Bromocriptine

Bromocriptine was proposed as an effective treatment for detrusor instability on the basis of one poorly designed and even more poorly analysed drug trial. At least three subsequent studies have shown the drug to be ineffective in the management of the unstable bladder.

Prostaglandin synthetase inhibitors

The role of prostaglandins in normal lower urinary tract function is unclear. Various prostaglandins can produce detrusor contraction *in vitro*. Of these PGF2α appears to be the most potent. Prostaglandin-mediated contractions are of slower onset and longer duration than those produced by acetylcholine. These findings led to trials of prostaglandin synthesis inhibitors in the management of detrusor instability. Cardozo *et al.* showed that flurbiprofen produced a significant reduction in incontinence episodes when compared to placebo. However, there were no significant differences in urodynamic parameters. Almost half of the patients had side-effects while on flurbiprofen. In another study, indomethacin failed to reduce the number of incontinence episodes. Again, around half of the patients had side-effects while on the non-steroidal anti-inflammatory drug. These drugs currently have no place in the management of detrusor instability.

The effect of a wide variety of other drugs on detrusor instability has been studied (Table 2). Some have been widely used in the management of incontinence, some are just starting to be evaluated, and others have been tried and found wanting. The literature on these drugs is limited and there is as yet no good reason to believe that any of them are superior to agents such as oxybutynin. Among the drugs which have been studied are:

Table 2 Drug treatment of incontinence

Drugs for the over-active detrusor
Propantheline (anticholinergic)
Emepromium bromide (anticholinergic)
Terodiline (anticholinergic and calcium antagonist)
Oxybutynin (anticholinergic and smooth muscle relaxant)
Dicyclomine (anticholinergic and smooth muscle relaxant)
Flavoxate (smooth muscle relaxant)
Flunarazine (calcium antagonist)
Flurbiprofen (prostaglandin inhibitor)
Imipramine (tricyclic antidepressant)
Doxepin (tricyclic antidepressant)
Baclofen (polysynaptic inhibitor)
Desmopressin (anti diuretic hormone analogue)
Bromocriptine
Terbutaline (β-adrenoceptor stimulator)
Verapamil (calcium antagonist)
Nifedipine (calcium antagonist)
Pinocidil (antihypertensive agent which opens potassium channels in vascular smooth
    muscle thereby hyperpolarizing the cell and reducing the effect of exitatory agents)

Propiverine hydrochloride (anticholinergic and calcium antagonist)
Clenobterol (β-2 sympathomimetric)

Drugs for genuine stress incontinence
Oestrogens
Ephedrine (α-adrenergic agonist)
Norfenefrine
Pseudo-ephedrine (α-adrenergic agonist)
Phenylpropanolamine (α-adrenergic agonist)

Drugs and the under-active detrusor
Intravesical prostaglandins
Bethanechol
Carbachol

Conclusions

The use of drugs in the management of detrusor instability and detrusor hyperreflexia is far from satisfactory. Although they may reduce the frequency of micturition, reduce the number of incontinence episodes, increase the volume of bladder filling at which unstable contractions occur, increase bladder capacity and reduce the height of unstable contractions, they rarely lead to continence when used by themselves. Their use is usually combined with a voiding regime, either regular timed voiding or bladder drill. They may also be combined with permanent catheterization or intermittent self-catheterization where involuntary contractions lead to leakage around the catheter or incontinence in the intervals between self-catheterization. Oxybutynin and imipramine are currently this author's drugs of choice. If these fail there seems little point in trying the alternatives.

Drugs and genuine stress incontinence

Oestrogens and α-adrenergic agents are currently used in the non-surgical management of females with genuine stress incontinence. The belief that oestrogens have an influence on lower urinary tract function is based on the common embryological origin of the bladder trigone, urethra and vagina and on the identification of oestrogen receptors in the female urethra where they are concentrated in the distal urethra. Among their effects are an increased density and sensitivity of α-adrenergic receptors and improvement in the mucosal seal mechanism by causing mucosal proliferation. There is controversy over the place of oestrogens in the management of incontinence, particularly genuine stress incontinence. Studies have shown that oestrogens increase maximul urethral pressure but have failed to show consistent benefit from using oestrogens in genuine stress incontinence. Indeed, most studies have shown oestrogens to be no better than placebo. Oestrogens have been more effective in improving the symptom of urgency. In view of the potential side-effects, including the increased risk of endometrial carcinoma, oestrogens should probably be avoided in the management of genuine stress incontinence. They have their place in the management of patients with symptoms due to atrophic urethritis. These atrophic changes in the mucosa of the lower urinary tract will be reflected in the vaginal mucosa.

Alpha-adrenergic agents are also used in the management of genuine stress incontinence. Stimulation of the α-adrenergic receptors in the bladder neck by drugs such as phenylpropanolamine, norfenefrine and ephedrine leads to an increase in maximual urethral pressure. The drugs are effective in patients with mild to moderate stress incontinence but are of little benefit for severe genuine stress incontinence. They have been used, with effect, in male patients with post-prostatectomy stress incontinence. Although usually well-tolerated, they may have significant side-effects, including elevation of blood pressure, palpitations, anxiety, tremor and headache. Their use is contraindicated in patients with hypertension, ischaemic heart disease and thyrotoxicosis. These drugs may be effective in patients with mild to moderate genuine stress incontinence but their use has to be balanced against the possibility of serious side-effects.

Although oestrogens alone are of no proven benefit in the management of genuine stress incontinence, the combination of an oestrogen and an α-adrenergic agent seems to be effective.

Drugs and the under-active detrusor

Based on our understanding of lower urinary tract physiology, two groups of drugs have been introduced for the management of the under-active detrusor: cholinergic agents and prostaglandins.

Cholinergic agents

Bethanechol chloride is a muscarinic agent resistant to degradation by acetylcholine. It has been in clinical use for over 50 years and has been the drug of choice for the promotion of bladder emptying. Although it is undoubtedly effective *in vitro* at causing bladder contraction, recent studies have cast doubt upon its clinical efficacy. Thus authors, such as Wein *et al.* and Barrett, were unable to demonstrate any facilitation of voiding in normal women or women with voiding disorders but without evidence of neurological disease or bladder outlet obstruction. In a recent review of the literature Finkbeiner concluded that, although pharmacologically active *in vitro* and *in vivo*, bethanechol chloride has not been shown to be clinically effective in promoting bladder emptying, regardless of the dose used, the route of administration or the disease state for which it was being used. Side-effects include nausea, vomiting, blurred vision, bradycardia and abdominal pain. Similar agents tried in an attempt to promote bladder emptying include the muscarinic agent carbachol which has to be given subcutaneously, and the anticholinesterase distigmine bromide which can be given orally or intramuscularly.

Prostaglandins

Prostaglandins, PGE, PGE2, PGF1α and PGF2α cause detrusor contraction. Of these, PGF2α is the most potent. The response of the detrusor to prostaglandins develops more slowly and is much more prolonged than the response to acetylcholines. They have to be given by intravesical installation or as a urethral jelly. When used clinically in the management of patients with voiding disorders they are absorbed through the mucosa. They appear to be effective in restoring normal bladder function in female patients with post-operative retention. These are patients without pre-operative voiding problems. The long-term results in patients with chronic urinary retention are variable and their place in management remains controversial. Side-effects include intestinal colic and dysmenorrhoea-like uterine cramps.

Other agents with proven *in vitro* effects on detrusor contraction include histamine, 5-hydroxytryptamine, vasoactive intestinal polypeptide and adenosine triphosphate. They have at present no clinical application.

References

Barrett DM. The effect of oral bethanecol chloride on voiding in female patients with excessive residual urine: a randomised double-blind study. *J. Urol.* 1981; **126:** 640–642.

Blaivis JG, Labib KB, Michalik SJ, Zayed AH. Cystometric response to propantheline in detrusor hyperreflexia: therapeutic implications. *J. Urol.* 1980; **124:** 259–262.

Cardozo LD, Stanton SL, Robinson H, Hole D. Evaluation of flurbiprofen in detrusor instability. *Br. Med. J.* 1980; **280:** 281–282.

Castleden CM, Duffin HM, Asher MJ, Yeomanson CW. Factors influencing outcome in elderly patients with urinary incontinence and detrusor instability. *Age Ageing* 1985; **14:** 303–307.

Castleden CM, Duffin HM, Golati RS. Double blind study of imipramine and placebo for incontinence due to bladder instability. *Age Ageing* 1986; **15:** 299–303.

Finkbeiner AE. Is bethanecol chloride clinically effective in promoting bladder emptying? A literature review. *J. Urol.* 1985; **134:** 443–448.

Mayhoff HH, Gerstenberg TC, Nordling J. Placebo—the drug of choice in female motor urge incontinence? *Br. J. Urol.* 1983; **55:** 34–37.

Moore KH, Hay DM, Imrie AE, Watson A. Goldstein M. Oxybutynin hydrochloride in the treatment of women with idiopathic detrusor instability. *Br. J. Urol.* 1990; **66:** 479–485.

Ouslander JG, Blausterin J, Connor A, Orzeck S, Yong CL. Pharmacokinetics and clinical effects of oxybutynin in geriatric patients. *J. Urol.* 1988; **140:** 47–50.

Robinson JM, Brocklehurst JC. Emepromium bromide and flavoxate hydrochloride in the treatment of urinary incontinence associated with detrusor instability in elderly women. *Br. J. Urol.* 1983; **55:** 371–376.

Tammela T, Kontturi M, Kaar K, Lukkarinen O. Intravesical prostaglandin F2 for promoting bladder emptying after surgery for female stress incontinence. *Br. J. Urol.* 1987; **60:** 43–46.

Tapp A, Fall M, Norgaard J, Massey A, Choa R, Carr T, Korhonen M, Abrams P. Terodiline: a dose titrated multi-centre study of the treatment of idiopathic detrusor instability in women. *J. Urol.* 1989; **142:** 1027–1031.

Thuroff JW, Bunke B, Ebner A *et al*. Randomised double-blind multicentre trial on treatment of frequency, urgency and incontinence related to detrusor hyperactivity: oxybutynin versus propantheline versus placebo. *J. Urol.* 1991; **145:** 813–817.

Wiseman PA, Malone-Lee J, Rai GS. Terodiline with bladder retraining for treating detrusor instability in elderly people. *Br. Med. J.* 1991; **302:** 994–996.

Wein AJ, Malloy TR, Shofer F, Raezar DM. The effects of bethanecol chloride on urodynamic parameters in normal women and in women with significant residual urine volumes. *J. Urol.* 1980; **124:** 397–399.

Zorzitto ML, Holliday PJ, Jewett MAS, Herschorn S, Fernie GR. Oxybutynin chloride for geriatric urinary dysfunction; a double blind placebo controlled trial. *Age Ageing* 1989; **18:** 195–200.

Chapter 7 _____

Surgical treatment of incontinence

Surgery remains the most effective therapeutic intervention for female patients with genuine stress incontinence and male patients with detrusor instability secondary to outflow tract obstruction. It is the treatment of last resort for those with idiopathic detrusor instability or detrusor hyperreflexia.

In elderly men with incontinence as a consequence of outflow obstruction, surgery is usually justified by the need to relieve outflow obstruction. Referring elderly women with genuine stress incontinence for surgery is a more difficult decision. The high probability of surgical cure has to be balanced against the risks of surgery. The patient's age, mental state and physical health will obviously influence any decision regarding surgery.

Surgery for genuine stress incontinence

Patients with genuine stress incontinence fall into two groups. In over 90 per cent the problem is anatomical. The sphincter mechanism is intact but because the proximal urethra is no longer an intra-abdominal organ any rise in intra-abdominal pressure is transmitted to the bladder but not to the proximal urethra. This may result in a transient reversal of the usual pressure gradient leading to stress incontinence. Surgery in these patients aims to re-position the bladder neck and proximal urethra in the abdominal pressure zone. This should result in a non-obstructive bladder neck in a non-mobile high retropubic position. The remaining 10 per cent of patients have Type III stress continence. Here there is damage to the sphincter mechanism as a result of surgery, radiation or pelvic fracture. These may lead to a rigid scarred urethra incapable of being compressed. Type III stress incontinence may also result from damage to the neural supply of the proximal urethra. Although the proximal urethra is correctly positioned, adequate transmission of pressure alterations to the urethra is impossible. Patients often have almost continuous incontinence, in addition to stress incontinence. The aim of surgery in these patients is to increase urethral resistance.

Over a hundred different surgical techniques for the management of genuine stress incontinence have been described. They fall into three main groups, the operations in each group being technical variations on the original operation. The three groups are (1) vaginal surgery, (2) suprapubic surgery, and (3) combined vaginal and suprapubic surgery.

In addition to these operations other procedures have been introduced that compress the urethra in patients with Type III stress incontinence. These include Teflon injections, the use of artificial sphincters and sling operations. Sling operations not only compress the proximal urethra but also elevate the bladder neck. As well as being used in Type III stress incontinence sling operations are also used in the treatment of patients where previous combined vaginal and suprapubic surgery has failed.

Whether or not patients who have detrusor instability in addition to genuine stress incontinence should be operated upon remains a matter of controversy. Some surgeons have reported good results regardless of the presence of detrusor instability and do not allow the presence or absence of unstable contractions to influence their decisions regarding surgery. Others have reported a marked reduction in surgical success rates in patients with co-existent detrusor instability. Since it is important not to operate on those whose stress incontinence is due to detrusor instability alone, pre-operative urodynamic studies of all patients being considered for surgery are necessary.

Vaginal surgery

The vaginal approach to the treatment of genuine stress incontinence is easy and associated with a low level of morbidity. Unfortunately, operations like anterior colporrhaphy are relatively ineffective at elevating the bladder neck and long-term success rates are less than 50 per cent. Through a midline anterior vaginal incision mattress sutures are placed at the bladder neck and along the proximal urethra to plicate the periurethral tissues.

Retropubic surgery

Although more difficult and having a higher morbidity than the transvaginal approach, suprapubic bladder neck suspensions like that originally described by Marshall, Marchetti and Krantz, have a reported success rate of over 90 per cent. The bladder neck and urethra are anchored to the back of the pubis and maintained in an intra-abdominal position by sutures between the periurethral area at the bladder neck and the pubic periosteum. They do not provide support behind the urethra. Complications include the development of osteitis pubis, wound infections and urethral obstruction due to kinking. Periurethral fibrosis may involve the urethra and lead to Type III stress incontinence. The Burch colposuspension has a number of advantages over the Marshall–Marchetti–Krantz operation. Urethral obstruction is rare and a moderately sized cystocele can be corrected at the same time.

Combined transvaginal and retropubic procedures

Combined transvaginal and retropubic procedures usually involve the use of needles to pass sutures from the vagina to the abdominal wall. Techniques such as those described by and named after Pereyra and Stamey are now the most commonly performed operations for the management of genuine stress incontinence. They have a reported cure rate in excess of 90 per cent.

Elderly patients tolerate these operations well, providing they are properly selected; success rates are lower than in younger age groups.

Sling operations

Sling operations are used in the management of Type III stress incontinence and in patients who have had failed combined transvaginal and retropubic surgery. These operations elevate the bladder neck and increase urethral resistance. The slings are normally formed from rectal fascia but can also be made from fascia lata, porcine skin, nylon or silastic. The sling is passed around the urethra and fixed to the pubic bone or rectus sheath. It elevates, supports and compresses the urethra. Cure rates of over 80 per cent are claimed—very good when one considers that these are very difficult cases.

Teflon injections

In Type III stress incontinence, urethral resistance can be increased by injecting inert materials like Teflon, a pyrolysed polytetrafluorethylene, or collagen into the urethra and periurethral tissues. The particles stimulate the ingrowth of fibroblasts and become encapsulated by a fibrous reaction. This results in permanent bolstering of the urethra. Early post-operative results are good but later results are less impressive. The operation can be done as an out-patient procedure under local anaesthesia. It is useful for the very elderly and those who are poor surgical risks. These injections have also been used in the management of post-prostatectomy stress incontinence due to sphincter damage. Here the results are poorer than in females, with only a quarter of the patients improving.

Artificial sphincters

Type III stress incontinence can also be managed using an artificial sphincter. These devices are also used in male patients with post-prostatectomy sphincter damage. The surgery is technically complex, with good results coming from specialized centres. In males with post-prostatectomy sphincter damage the device consists of a circular cuff placed around the bulbar urethra, an inflate/deflate pump placed in the scrotum and a fluid-filled reservoir beneath the rectus abdominis fascia. Although success rates of over 70 per cent are claimed, many patients require further surgery because of mechanical problems.

Surgery and the unstable bladder

There are two surgical approaches to the management of the unstable bladder. The first, and more successful, is to relieve outflow obstruction in male patients with detrusor instability secondary to obstruction. The alternative approach, used in patients with idiopathic detrusor instability or detrusor hyperreflexia, is to interrupt the nerve supply to the bladder.

The relief of outflow obstruction

Bladder outflow obstruction is rare in the female. The relationship between outflow obstruction and detrusor instability which exists in the male does not seem to occur in the female. Where outflow obstruction and detrusor instability do co-exist in the female, relief of the obstruction rarely results in the bladder reverting to stability.

Outflow obstruction is much commoner in the male. Detrusor instability frequently develops in response to outflow obstruction and is often reversed when the obstruction is relieved. Over half of the patients who undergo prostatectomy have unstable bladders. Two-thirds of these revert to normal after relief of the obstruction, usually within 3–6 months. The prevalence of detrusor instability after relief of outflow obstruction by prostatic resection approximates to the natural prevalence for this age group; this probably accounts for the failure of all patients to benefit from surgery. The mortality rate for prostatectomy in patients over 70 years of age is near 1 per cent. The main contraindication is severe cognitive impairment.

Stents made of fine corrosion-resistant superalloy wire have been used in the past in the treatment of urethral strictures and dyssynergic sphincters. They are currently being evaluated as an alternative to prostatectomy in those who are unfit, and appear to be a safe and effective alternative.

Patients who fail to respond to surgery run the risk of worsening incontinence post-operatively because unstable contractions can more easily overcome the now normal outflow resistance. As discussed in an earlier chapter, the response of unstable contractions to intravesical lignocaine, or the duration of electrically evoked responses, are purported to identify which patients will have persistent detrusor instability post-operatively. This knowledge may not influence management. The relief of outflow obstruction may be necessary if other complications, including renal, vesical and prostatic infection, calculi and impaired renal function, are to be avoided.

Where patients have a neurological lesion in addition to outflow obstruction, it is impossible to know for certain if the urge incontinence is secondary to the obstruction or the neurological lesion. Obviously, if the patient's symptoms had their onset at the same time as they had a cerebrovascular accident it is likely that the incontinence is due to detrusor hyperreflexia. Usually the onset of a neurological lesion is less dramatic as in Parkinson's disease and dementia and the distinction is much more difficult to make. After prostatectomy almost half of these patients will remain incontinent or may be more incontinent. Unless the outflow obstruction is relieved, drugs with anticholinergic effects cannot safely be used because of the dangers of precipitating urinary retention.

Augmentation cystoplasty

Patients with idiopathic detrusor instability and detrusor hyperreflexia who are refractory to medical treatment pose a major therapeutic challenge for which there is as yet no satisfactory surgical solution. A variety of operations have been introduced for the management of these patients. Of these augmentation cystoplasty, also known as a clam cystoplasty, is currently the most popular. The operation involves the bladder being almost completely bivalved in the coronal plane, giving it the appearance of an open clam. A length of ileum with its own blood supply is then sutured to the bladder. The circular fibres of the bowel segment are transected to improve compliance and to protect against mass contractions of the bowel segment. Ileum is preferred to colon as there is less risk of malignant change. Bladder capacity is increased and the presence of the cystoplasty makes involuntary contractions ineffective. It may also compromise the efficacy of voluntary detrusor contractions.

Post-operatively most patients have to strain in order to void. Some will be unable to void adequately by straining alone and need a bladder neck incision or Otis sphincterotomy. Even after reducing outflow resistance, around a third of patients require intermittent self-catheterization. In effect, one lower urinary tract dysfunction has been replaced by another which is easier to manage. All patients continue voiding mucus and in some this will form into marble-shaped balls which may need to be removed endoscopically. Other complications include fistula formation, urinary tract infection, mild acid–base disturbance, late perforation and risk of malignant change. Satisfactory outcomes have been reported in over 80 per cent of patients. This is a major operation with significant complications. There are no reports on its use in the elderly and even in the young it remains a treatment of last resort reserved for those with disabling symptoms who have failed to respond to more conservative management.

Selective sacral neurectomy

A variety of different operations have been developed over the years with the common aim of denervating the bladder. Their introduction and subsequent fall from favour is an indication of their limited efficacy. In interrupting the neural supply they may, if effective, produce an acontractile bladder rather than one which functions normally.

Selective sacral neurectomy involves denervating the bladder by transection of the second, third or fourth sacral nerve roots exposed via a limited sacral laminectomy. The level for transection is selecting by combining information obtained from pre-operative nerve root blocks and intra-operative nerve stimulation. In practice, it is usually the third sacral nerve root which is transected. Surgery aims to produce an increase in bladder capacity, a decrease in detrusor hyperreflexia and an unchanged sphincter mechanism. Most studies on the effectiveness of this operation have involved small numbers of patients. Although most have reported symptomatic improvement in the majority of patients, most of these have had persistent detrusor instability. At best only half of the patients gain long-term symptomatic relief. Selective sacral neurectomy has not been used in the elderly and even in the young there are differing views as to whether or not it has a place in the management of incontinence.

Subtrigonal phenol injection

Subtrigonal phenol injection is another operation where poor long-term results have dampened initial enthusiasm. The operation aims to destroy the pelvic plexus where it lies on the anterolateral vaginal wall. This involves injecting a 6.5% solution of aqueous phenol through a point half-way between the ureteric orifice and the internal urethral meatus on each side. The needle is introduced under cystoscopic control and inserted to a depth of 2–3 cm. More aqueous phenol is introduced on each side via a transvulval route to denervate the lower trigonal region which may escape the initial injection. The main advantage of this procedure is its relative simplicity and the fact that patients can be treated as day cases. It is contraindicated in male patients as it may lead to impotence. Initial reports claimed significant symptomatic and urodynamic improvement in two-thirds of patients but a significant minority develop urinary retention and have to be taught intermittent self-catheterization. Other complications include lower ureteric stricture, bladder fistula and femoral nerve palsy. Beneficial results are usually transient: in females the success rate at one month is 48 per cent falling to 16 per cent at 6 months. The short duration of any benefit and the risks involved, including those associated with general anaesthesia, mean that it can no longer be recommended.

Bladder transection

Transection of the detrusor muscle in a line 2 cm above the interureteric bar, across the back of the bladder and extending on each side to a point 2 cm proximal to the bladder neck anteriorly with an incision through the mucosa and muscle, has also been used in the management of detrusor instability. This results in division of the intramural parasympathetic nerves and also in disruption of the anatomical and myoelectrical continuity of the detrusor. Although symptomatic improvement in 50–75 per cent of patients has been claimed, most patients continue to have persistent instability. Reported series have contained mainly patients with idiopathic detrusor instability. It is tempting to conclude that much of the symptomatic improvement in these patients represents a placebo response.

Bladder distension

Bladder distension is yet another technique introduced in an effort to cure surgically detrusor instability and hyperreflexia. A specially designed balloon tied over a Foley catheter is inserted into the bladder and inflated with saline by connecting the catheter to an intravenous drip set. The height of the drip bottle above the bladder is kept equivalent to the patient's systolic blood pressure. The balloon is kept inflated for 2 hours but is emptied for 5 minutes in each half-hour. A modification of this technique is to use a Cystomat, a disposable apparatus for bladder irrigation, to distend the bladder continuously for a week. The aim of this technique is to produce ischaemic and mechanical damage to nerve terminals and muscle fibres. Results are usually poor and complications include bladder rupture.

With the exception of surgery to relieve outflow obstruction and possibly of clam cystoplasty in exceptional circumstances, none of the above operations has a place in the routine management of detrusor instability or hyperreflexia in the elderly.

Surgical management of detrusor sphincter dyssynergia

Detrusor sphincter dyssynergia is nearly always due to a neurological lesion of the spinal cord. The surgical treatment of this is a transurethral external sphincterotomy. Patients are generally incontinent post-operatively. An alternative means of management is to combine the use of anticholinergic agents to make the bladder atonic with intermittent self-catheterization. If anticholinergics fail to lead to an atonic bladder, clam cystoplasty can be combined with intermittent self-catheterization.

References

Abrams PH, Farrar DJ, Turner-Warwick RT, Whiteside CJ, Feneley RCL. The results of prostatectomy: a symptomatic and urodynamic analysis of 152 patients. *J. Urol.* 1979; **121:** 640–642.

Bramble FJ. The clam cystoplasty. *Br. J. Urol.* 1990; **66:** 337–341.

Deane AM, English P, Hehir M, Williams JP, Worth PHL. Teflon injection in stress incontinence. *Br. J. Urol.* 1985; **57:** 78–80.

Eastwood HDH, Smart CJ. Urinary incontinence in the disabled elderly male. *Age Ageing* 1985; **14:** 235–239.

Lucas MG, Thomas DG, Clarke S, Forster DMC. Long-term follow-up of selective sacral neurectomy. *Br. J. Urol.* 1988; **61:** 218–220.

Mundy AR. The surgical treatment of urge incontinence of urine. *J. Urol.* 1982; **128:** 481–483.

Pengelly AW, Stevenson DP, Milroy EJG, Whiteside CJ, Turner-Warwick RT. Results of prolonged bladder distension as treatment for detrusor instability. *Br. J. Urol.* 1978; **50:** 243–245.

Rosenbaum TP, Shaw JR, Worth PHL. Transtrigonal phenol failed the test of time. *Br. J. Urol.* 1990; **66:** 164–169.

Stanton SL, Cardozo LD. Surgical treatment of incontinence in elderly women. *Surg., Gynaecol. Obstet.* 1980; **150:** 555–557.

Chapter 8

Other aspects of management

The management of urinary incontinence in elderly patients generally involves the simultaneous use of a number of different treatment strategies, some of which have already been reviewed. Among the other options available are physiotherapy, environmental manipulation, catheters, electronic aids and protective garments. Here the emphasis is on those aspects of these treatments which are of interest to physicians. Less attention is paid to some of the more practical aspects of their use which are primarily of interest to nursing and paramedical staff.

Physiotherapy

Physiotherapy is a widely used, effective and safe way of managing female patients with genuine stress incontinence. It may be used as a first-line treatment or as an alternative to surgery in those who are unfit for surgery or who decline its use. It is occasionally useful in male patients with post-prostatectomy incontinence due to sphincter damage. Although its efficacy is well-established there remain a number of unresolved questions regarding its use. What is the most effective regime? Which patients are most likely to benefit? Does a perineometer improve results? Does the addition of electrical therapy improve results? What is the place of vaginal cones?

The purpose of pelvic floor exercises is to increase the tone and power of the periurethral striated muscles thereby improving urethral closure and enhancing urethral support. Contraction of these muscles does not come naturally to many women and around 40 per cent are unable to contract them properly without prior instruction. It is thus important that the physiotherapists perform a vaginal examination to assess the patient's ability to contract these muscles and, where necessary, to educate her in their use. The commonest mistake made by patients is to exercise their gluteal muscles instead of the periurethral pelvic floor muscles. The patient is shown a variety of exercises, for example, while lying on her back with her legs stretched out and crossed at the ankles to squeeze her thighs together and then pull up inside. It should be noted that interrupting the flow of urine during micturition gives a measure of progress but is not, of itself, a useful exercise.

With a large number of regimes described in the literature there seems to be no consensus on how often the exercises should be done, the number of contractions to be performed on each occasion, or the duration of each contraction. In some studies patients have exercised once a day, performing a hundred contractions at the one time. Others have been instructed to perform five contractions every half hour. Between these extremes are a variety of regimes. The duration of the pelvic floor contraction has also varied widely, from as short as two seconds to as long as half a minute.

The variation in the regimes used may account for some of the variability in the reported efficacy of this form of treatment. In most studies the majority of patients have improved although only a minority of these are cured. In general, around two-thirds of patients are cured or improved. This grouping of those who are cured and those who improve may give a false idea of the overall efficacy of physiotherapy. Usually less than half of the patients are cured or sufficiently improved to decide that they do not require surgery. Although surgery is much more effective in leading to a cure it is not without its risks, whereas physiotherapy is without known complications.

While some authors have found that the elderly and those with severe stress incontinence respond poorly to physiotherapy, others have failed to identify any difference in response rates. Even if physiotherapy were less effective in the elderly or in those with severe incontinence it would still seem reasonable to try it on all patients before considering surgery.

Whether or not a perineometer improves results is also unclear. This consists of a cuffed vaginal catheter connected to a manometer. It allows the patient to measure the strength of her pelvic floor contractions and thus to monitor her progress, i.e. it acts as a form of feedback. While some authors have found that patients using a perineometer do better than those not using one, others have failed to detect any difference in outcome.

Electrical therapy may be used alone or as an adjunct to pelvic floor exercises. The aim is to provide the maximum muscle contraction with the minimum sensory discomfort. Electrical therapy is said to improve the blood supply to muscles, to break down any adhesions which may be present and to increase muscle tone. A major effect is to contract the pelvic floor muscles and thus give the patient an awareness of how they contract, thereby improving her ability to contract them voluntarily.

Faradism in which a low-frequency current is used was the original form of electrical therapy but has been superseded by interferential therapy. This involves the application to the body of two slightly different but medium-frequency alternating currents. This gives a low-frequency effect in the tissues equal to the difference between the two medium-frequency currents, enabling the current to penetrate deeper as it overcomes the high skin resistance to low-frequency currents. The current is delivered by pads or suction cups. Two or four electrodes may be used. If two are used one electrode is placed under the ischiael tuberosity and the second over the anterior perineum. It is a non-invasive procedure which can be used by itself, for example in elderly people unable to perform pelvic floor exercises or as an adjunct to pelvic floor exercises. Interferential therapy may also have a place in the management of patients with detrusor instability. Contraction of pelvic floor muscles leads to reflex inhibition of the detrusor muscle. This reflex is mediated by afferents from muscle stretch receptors travelling in the pudendal nerve. Electrical stimulation of the pudendal nerve has the same effect. It remains to be shown whether or not this form of therapy will have a place in clinical practice.

Another method of re-educating pelvic floor muscles is the use of cones. This involves having the patient retain cones of increasing weight in her vagina for around 15 minutes a couple of times a day. When she can manage to retain a cone on two consecutive occasions she progresses to the next weight. The use of cones appears to be at least as effective as routine pelvic floor exercises. It has one major advantage: professional time taken to educate patients in the use of cones is less than that required for routine pelvic floor exercises making it much more cost effective. Cones, however, are not suitable for all patients.

Catheters

In the management of incontinent patients the insertion of an indwelling catheter is usually considered to be the final therapeutic option, i.e. it is the treatment of last resort. Despite its negative image it may greatly improve the patient's quality of life. He or she is freed from the discomfort and embarrassment of wet clothes, the inconvenience of always needing to be near a toilet and the shame of polluting the environment of others. Similarly, carers are spared the staining of furniture, the smell of stale urine and the excess laundry requirements. While the insertion of a catheter may render some patients dry and greatly improve their quality of life, their use is not without its risks or problems. One of the commonest complications in the catheterized elderly population is bypassing of urine. The patient is incontinent of urine around the catheter. Not only does the patient remain wet but he or she now faces the additional problems that arise from having an indwelling catheter. Catheterization may be deemed necessary because voiding problems lead to urinary retention. Alternatively it may be used in a last-ditch effort to render the patient dry. In the latter case decisions regarding the introduction of a catheter and whether or not to persist with it are usually made by the patient, or if the patient is mentally impaired by those directly responsible for their care. Some relatives and care staff can only cope with an incontinent patient if they are rendered dry by the use of a catheter. Others find the catheter a daunting responsibility or consider it undignified and prefer to cope with the patient's incontinence.

External collecting devices

Satisfactory external collecting devices are only available for male patients. Despite much effort, none has yet been designed that copes with the female shape. They should be considered in all incontinent male patients but their use may lead to a number of complications, including urinary tract infections, urethral diverticulae or fistulae, skin ulceration and penile gangrene. Various models are available, for example, Conveen®, Bard® penile sheaths, Texas® catheter, Seton® incontinence sheath. These sheaths are usually left in position for up to 24 hours at a time. An alternative to the incontinence sheath is the pubic pressure urinal in which urine empties into a collecting urinal strapped around the waist.

Internal collecting devices

Catheters for the relief of urinary retention have been available for over five thousand years. Indwelling balloon catheters have been available since the middle of the last century. Closed drainage systems were first introduced in the 1950s. Before that time catheter tubes emptied into open bottles. Catheters can be classified according to their use:

(a) Simple penile catheters, e.g. Jaques® catheter. These have no self-retaining device and are used when the catheter is not to be left *in situ*.
(b) Self-retaining catheters, e.g. Foley® balloon catheter. This has two channels, the drainage tube and the conduit for the water used to fill the retaining balloon.
(c) Suprapubic catheters, e.g. Malecot®.

Catheter size is usually given in the French or Charriere's scale as circumference in millimetres. Most patients require Charriere 14–18. Most catheters in common use are male length (41 cm). Shorter female length catheters (23 cm) are also available. The capacity of the retaining balloon caries from 5 to 30 ml.

Catheters can also be classified according to the material from which they are made. This may be metal, silicone, latex, latex coated with silicone (Silastic) or latex coated with Teflon. Latex catheters have a thick wall relative to the size of the lumen. The surface is not very smooth. Silicone catheters and silicone- or Teflon-coated latex catheters have a smoother surface and are thus supposed to be associated with less encrustation. This claim, however, is controversial. They are undoubtedly associated with less urethral irritation and are also supposed to be longer lasting. They have a larger lumen relative to wall size than do latex catheters.

There are a large number of different collecting bags available and also a wide variety of different systems to support the bags. The bag may be held on the leg by latex straps. Alternatively it may be supported in a thigh pocket, for example the Brevet Netti® urine bag holder, or suspended from a waist belt, for example Seton® portabag and belt. It can also be held in the pocket of a pair of specially designed knickers, for example Brevet® cathepants. Leg bags are easy to attach to the calf where they are camouflaged by wearing trousers. Attaching them to the thigh is often unsatisfactory. If a skirt is being worn one of the other support systems is indicated. Larger capacity drainage bags are needed at night. This may be managed by changing the bag or by connecting a night bag to the day bag using a special connector, for example Lic connector. The advantage of the latter system is that the drainage system remains closed.

Complications and their management

The three main complications of long-term catheterization are infection, encrustation and bypassing. Other problems include bladder calculi and bladder neoplasm. Malignant change occurs in patients who have been catheterized for over 10 years, so this risk is not relevant to the catheterized elderly patient. Catheter blockage or leakage of urine around the catheter usually results in the catheter requiring replacement within a month. Repetitive catheter changes are associated with their own complications, including urethral erosion, the creation of false passages and stricture formation.

Infection

Before the introduction of closed drainage systems virtually all patients had significant bacteriuria within 4 days. With modern catheters most patients will have significant bacteriuria within a month. Thus it can be assumed that all patients permanently catheterized for the management of established incontinence will develop bacteriuria. Where short-term catheterization is used, bacteriuria develops most rapidly in the elderly, females and those with neuropathic bladder disorders. Bacteriuria and significant infection are not synonymous. Treatment is only indicated where there is evidence of systemic infection.

Infecting organisms arise predominantly from the lower gastrointestinal tract. They gain access to the bladder by three main routes: (1) they may travel up the urethra in the space between the catheter and the urethral wall; (2) they may enter the catheter system via the collecting bag which can become contaminated while the bag is being emptied; (3) they may enter via the junction between the catheter and the collecting bag which may become contaminated if disconnected for bladder irrigation or to change the bag at night.

Unless antibiotics have been used the bacteria found in the bladders of recently catheterized patients are similar to those causing urinary tract infections in the non-catheterized population. Thus *Escherichia coli* is the commonest pathogen. With the passage of time more unusual pathogenic organisms, such as *Morganella morganii*, can be found and with long-term catheterization the infection is usually polymicrobial. Attempts to prevent the development of bacteriuria by the use of antiseptic bladder washouts or local antibiotic therapy have met with mixed results. They probably have little, if any, beneficial effect. Indeed, breaking the closed drainage system to irrigate the bladder allows bacteria the opportunity to enter the bladder. More worrying is that their use may be associated with the development of resistant organisms. The use of systemic antibiotics to prevent bacteriuria is effective but only for as long as they are used. Once stopped the patient rapidly develops bacteriuria with organisms resistant to the antibiotic used. It is generally agreed that the presence of bacteriuria of itself is not an indication for antibiotic therapy, which should be reserved for patients with evidence of systemic infection. Approximately two-thirds of febrile episodes in elderly patients with catheters *in situ* arise in the urinary tract. Other infections which may occur in catheterized patients include purulent epididymitis, scrotal abscess, prostatic abscess and periurethral abscess formation.

Encrustation

Catheter encrustation is a common problem which may lead to catheter blockage. This is one of the three main problems which lead to a catheter change, the others are bypassing of urine and catheter rejection. It affects around half of those with long-term indwelling urethral catheters. Blockage may result in either bypassing of urine or retention. Encrustations form only on catheter surfaces which are exposed to urine. They are composed mainly of struvite (ammonium magnesium phosphate) and calcium phosphate with, as yet, uncharacterized organic components. In a minority of patients calcium oxalate is also present. There is a close correlation between the proportion of the encrustation material composed of calcium phosphate and the frequency of catheter blockage. Precipitation of struvite occurs in the alkaline urine of patients infected with urease-producing bacteria, such as *Proteus*, *Klebsiella* and *Pseudomonas*. However, not all patients infected with urease-producing organisms have problems with encrustation. Thus other factors are important.

Some patients seem to be more susceptible to encrustation than others. This differential susceptibility may be related to the presence of inhibitors of crystal formation in the urine. Silicone and silicone-coated catheters are supposed to be less susceptible to encrustation by virtue of their smoother surfaces but this has been challenged. It has been suggested that the conflicting reports of differing susceptibility to encrustation of different catheters is due to patient variation rather than the different characteristics of the catheters being assessed.

Prevention of catheter encrustation is primarily by the use of bladder washouts. Deposits are removed as a result of the physical forces involved rather than the chemical properties of the agent used. A possible exception is the use of acidic solutions, such as Suby G, which may also dissolve the crystals. The benefits gained by increasing catheter time *in situ* and thus reducing the number of catheter changes may be offset by the potential risks. There is an increased exfoliation of bladder mucosal cells and an increased risk of infection because of the repeated interruption of the closed drainage system.

Bypassing of urine

Bypassing of urine is a common complication of long-term catheterization in the elderly. Around 40 per cent of the catheterized elderly will leak urine around the catheter due either to catheter blockage, as discussed earlier, or involuntary bladder contractions. The latter are triggered by the catheter and its balloon. Where bypassing is due to involuntary contractions, initial management involves replacement of the catheter by one with a smaller calibre tube and a smaller capacity balloon. If this fails, drug therapy (e.g. oxybutynin) can be tried. Replacement with a larger catheter will irritate the bladder further and is counterproductive. Larger catheters may also block urethral glands with consequent infection.

Rejection of catheters

This appears to have two possible causes. The catheter may be forcibly pulled out by a confused patient. Alternatively, and more commonly, the catheter may be forcibly expelled by an involuntary detrusor contraction.

Intermittent self-catheterization

Intermittent self-catheterization has been used for over 20 years. It is widely used in the management of urinary retention, especially in patients with spinal injuries and is only effective where there is a significant residual volume of urine. Patients need to be well-motivated. Although requiring some dexterity, it has been mastered by many disabled patients and can also be mastered by the elderly. The technique is not sterile. The patient washes her hands and the periurethral area. A lubricant, for example KY jelly or lignocaine gel, is used. The catheter is inserted at least four times daily and changed every 2 weeks. The catheter is rinsed in tap water and then boiled for half a minute or immersed in 0.016% sodium hypochloride solution (Milton's solution) over night. Complications are rare, especially in females. Initially the majority of patients will have urethral bleeding, which can be expected to resolve spontaneously within a few weeks. Other complications include urethral stricture, epididymo-orchitis and bladder calculi.

Suprapubic catheterization

Suprapubic catheterization is only indicated where the urethra is blocked. Urethral catheters have a number of advantages over suprapubic catheters. They are easier to insert, easier to change and drain the bladder more efficiently. There is no difference in the rate of infection. Complications of suprapubic catheterization include infection, leakage and haematoma formation at the site of insertion.

Electronic aids

Electrical therapy has been used in the management of incontinence for over 25 years. Electrical stimulation of the pelvic floor muscles will directly increase intraurethral pressure. Stimulation of these muscles also leads to reflex inhibition of the detrusor muscle. This form of therapy has been used in the management of genuine stress incontinence, detrusor instability and hyperreflexia and post-prostatectomy incontinence.

The use of interferential therapy as an adjuct or alternative to physiotherapy in patients with genuine stress incontinence has already been discussed. Various other forms of electrical therapy have been and are being evaluated. Cutaneous electrodes can be attached to the perineum or inserted into the vagina or anal canal. Alternatively, implanted electrodes can be attached directly to sacral nerves. The appropriate nerves are identified pre-operatively by test stimulation. This surgery may be combined with dorsal rhizotomy and selective peripheral neurotomy to obtain the best results in patients with neuropathic bladder disorders. Electronic devices have also been developed in which the electrical stimulation is triggered by a rise in intravesical pressure.

Electrical therapy is usually reserved for patients who have failed to respond to more conservative measures. Success rates of 30–70 per cent have been claimed but this form of therapy is still being evaluated and has as yet no part to play in the routine management of incontinent elderly patients. It is doubtful if it will become an acceptable or practical form of therapy in this age group in the foreseeable future.

Protective garments

With appropriate investigation and management some incontinent elderly patients will be cured and many more improved. There will, however, remain patients who need special garments to protect themselves, their clothes and their environment. As with catheterization, the use of protective garments should be reserved for those patients who have failed to respond adequately to other forms of treatment. Unfortunately, protective garments are often the first and only form of treatment used. Many patients resort to their use without prior medical or nursing consultation. Around two-thirds of the incontinent elderly in the community use incontinence aids, absorbent pads being the most popular. Many women use menstrual products or home-made pads, which is unsatisfactory when there are easily obtainable specially designed pant and pad systems. The purpose of these systems is to soak up urine thus keeping the patient comfortable while at the same time protecting their clothes and furniture.

Most of the published work in this area has involved the assessment of two systems, Kanga® pants and Molynycke® pants and pads. The parts are washable and the pads disposable. The Kanga system was developed in the late 1960s. Originally called Marsupial pants, they are designed for use when patients are out of bed. The pants are made of 100 per cent knitted polyester, which looks and feels like cotton and is permeable and non-absorbable. A waterproof pouch made of knitted nylon coated with polyurethane is sewn to the outside. This pouch starts just below the umbilicus and continues over the perineum to the back. The absorbent pads, made of 100 per cent cellulose, are folded double before being inserted into the pouch. The idea is that urine passes through the pants into the pad and provided the pad is changed before it becomes saturated with urine the patient's skin will remain reasonably dry. The waterproof pouch protects the patient's clothes and environment. The pads are changed without needing to remove the pants. Kanga pants come in a variety of sizes and designs. When the standard Kanga pant is used the pads should be placed anteriorly in the pouch over the penile area in males and over the perineum in females. Male and female pants with the whole pouch appropriately sited are also available. The pants should each last about a year.

Molynycke pants are made of elasticated Helanca thread knitted with loose stitches. There are two Lycra ribbons to hold the pads in place. The pants are elastic and one size is expected to fit all patients. They should last at least 2 months. The pads, which are worn inside the pants, have an upper surface of non-woven material allowing urine through and thus keeping the skin dry. The absorbent material is cellulose pulp and the pad is backed with waterproof polyethylene.

Both systems are satisfactory. The Kanga pants cannot be used if the patient is also incontinent of faeces, while the Molynycke system is not contraindicated in this situation. Even when pads fail to contain all the urine lost the amount of urine getting on to the patient's clothes and on to furniture is greatly reduced.

Special protective sheets are available for use when the patient is in bed. The design of these is similar to that of pads, i.e. a hydrophobic surface membrane, an absorptive vegetable fibre and a waterproof base. The popular Kylie absorbent bed sheet consists of an upper layer of hydrophobic brushed nylon, through which the urine passes to a middle hydrophilic layer made of rayon, which lies on a waterproof layer.

Various other incontinence aids are available. If odour is a problem, there are neutralizing deodorants which help eliminate smell, e.g. Nilodor®. Smell can also be reduced by paying attention to the patient's personal cleanliness and changing wet clothes as speedily as possible. Special clothes can be obtained. For example, trousers with extra-long flies to facilitate the use of a bottle or skirts which open at the back for chair-fast patients.

Functional aspects and environmental manipulation

When assessing and treating incontinent elderly patients, attention should be paid to the patient's functional status. Improving mobility in patients with Parkinson's disease or cerebrovascular disease may improve continence by allowing a patient with urgency to reach the toilet before being incontinent. Successful treatment of a toxic confusional state or faecal impaction may have equally dramatic effects. Where possible, drugs with an adverse effect on the bladder should be reduced or stopped.

The patient's environment may also need altering. Providing a bedside commode or urine bottle may improve nocturnal continence. Toilets in residential homes, nursing homes and hospitals should be appropriately sited. They should also be signposted, adequately marked and adapted for disabled people. Suitable adaptations may be needed in the toilet for patients living in their own homes.

When dealing with the incontinent elderly, therapeutic options may be limited because of cognitive impairment, physical disability or advanced age. At the same time management often needs to be multifaceted. In an elderly lady with an uninhibited neuropathic bladder secondary to a cerebrovascular accident, management may involve a toileting regime, the use of drugs, physiotherapy to improve her mobility, the use of appropriate protective garments and environmental manipulation.

References

Castelden CM, Duffin HM, Mitchell EP. The effect of physiotherapy on stress incontinence. *Age Ageing* 1984; **13**: 235–237.

Ferrie BG, Glen ES, Hunter B. Long-term urethral catheter drainage. *Br. Med. J.* 1979; **2**: 1046–1047.

Getliffe, KA, Mulhall AB. The encrustation of indwelling catheters. *Br. J. Urol.* 1991; **67**: 337–341.

Hukins DWL, Hickey DS, Kennedy AP. Catheter encrustation by struvite. *Br. J. Urol.* 1983; **55**: 304–305.

Mouritsen L, Frimodt-Moller C, Moller M. Long-term effect of pelvic floor exercises on female urinary incontinence. *Br. J. Urol.* 1991; **68**: 32–37.

Sabanathan, K. Castelden CM, Mitchell CJ. The problem of bacteriuria with indwelling urethral catheterisation. *Age Ageing* 1985; **14**: 85–90.

Tanagho EA, Schmidt RA, Orvis BR. Neural stimulation for control of voiding dysfunction: a preliminary report in 22 patients with serious neuropathic voiding disorders. *J. Urol.* 1989; **142**: 340–345.

Whitelaw S, Hammonds JC, Tregelas R. Clean intermittent self-catheterisation in the elderly. *Br. J. Urol.* 1987; **60**: 125–127.

Chapter 9

Physiology of defecation

Before reviewing the pathophysiological mechanisms which lead to faecal incontinence it is necessary to consider the structures responsible for the maintenance of faecal continence. These are the puborectalis muscle, the internal anal sphincter, the external anal sphincter and the anal cushions.

Anatomy of the lower gastrointestinal tract

The main anatomical features are shown in Fig 11. The rectum differs from

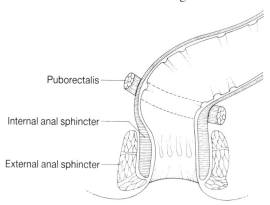

Puborectalis

Internal anal sphincter

External anal sphincter

Figure 11 Anatomy of the lower gastrointestinal tract.

the colon in that its outer longitudinal coat is evenly distributed around its surface; in the remainder of the colon it forms three distinct bands known as the Taeniae coli joined by a thin layer of longitudinal muscle. The rectum starts opposite the third part of the sacrum, passing downwards and forwards following the concavity of the sacrum and coccyx. It joins the anus at the anorectal ring. The anal canal extends downwards and backwards, its axis forming an angle of almost 90 degrees with that of the rectum. The angle between the rectum and anus is maintained by the puborectalis muscle. This muscle arises from the back of the pubic bone and loops around the anorectal junction to meet fibres from the other side forming a sling. Contraction of the puborectalis muscle draws the rectum upwards and forwards increasing the anorectal angle.

The circular smooth muscle coat of the lower 3 cm of the anal canal is over four times thicker than that of the lower rectum and forms the internal anal sphincter. This circular coat is surrounded by a thin layer of longitudinal muscle around which is a tube of striated muscle called the external anal sphincter. The terms internal and external anal sphincter do not imply that one lies superficial to the other but refer to the fact that one lies internal to and thus is surrounded by the other, i.e. a tube within a tube. The external anal sphincter fuses with the puborectalis muscle and these two muscles tend to act as a unit.

The lower part of the anal canal is lined by modified stratified squamous epithelium, while the upper end is lined by columnar epithelium with tubular glands. The anal canal has an extremely rich nerve supply. It is sensitive to touch, pain, heat and cold and can distinguish flatus from liquid or solid faeces. The sensory fibres travel in the pudendal nerve. Rectal distension produces a feeling of fullness in the perineum which may be associated with a feeling of impending evacuation. The receptors mediating this sensation do not appear to be in the rectum itself as the sensation remains if the rectum is removed and the colon is anastomosed to the upper anal canal. It may be that changes in rectal volume are detected by stretch receptors in the levator ani muscle. The internal anal sphincter receives its motor supply from the sympathetic and parasympathetic systems. The sympathetic supply comes via the hypogastric nerves from the fifth lumbar segment. The parasympathetic supply is via the nervi erigentes from the first to third sacral segments. The puborectalis and the external sphincter are supplied by the pudendal nerve and by the perineal branch of the fourth sacral nerve.

The maintenance of continence

The rectum acts as a reservoir for the storage of faeces which are then expelled when the time is socially convenient.

Internal anal sphincter

The internal anal sphincter is maintained in a state of near-maximum contraction. Its main reflex activity is to relax, which it does in response to rectal distension. This is the rectosphincteric reflex and it is believed to be an intramural reflex mediated by the myenteric and submucosal plexuses. It is still present in patients with lesions of the spinal cord, cauda equina and sacral roots but absent in those with Hirschsprung's disease. The internal sphincter is the main contributor to the resting anal tone. Maximum pressure is found half way along the internal sphincter. It prevents leakage of the small amount of faeces which enters the rectum but is insufficient to distend it to a level which results in reflex relaxation of the internal sphincter.

The external anal sphincter

The external anal sphincter, like the internal anal sphincter, is in a state of continuous contraction. It is usually maintained at a low level of contraction and contracts continuously, even during sleep. The afferent limb of the spinal cord reflex responsible for keeping it in a state of continuous contraction probably arises in the muscle itself. In patients with tabes dorsalis the afferent limb is lost and there is no resting electrical activity in the muscle. Voluntary contraction is still possible as the efferent limb is preserved.

Unlike the internal sphincter the external sphincter responds to a number of different stimuli. It contracts more vigorously in response to rises in intra-abdominal pressure as on coughing, sneezing or lifting and thus acts as a protective mechanism in these situations. Where the rise in intra-abdominal pressure is associated with the act of defecation the external sphincter relaxes. It contracts more vigorously in response to rectal distension. However, over-distension of the rectum causes it to relax. It will contract more vigorously in response to perianal stimulation (the anal reflex). In addition to these reflex responses, the external sphincter is also under voluntary control. Voluntary contraction can only be maintained for about 60 seconds. If the external sphincter is divided, continence is maintained providing the puborectalis remains intact. The main contribution of the external sphincter to continence is in resisting leakage where there are transient rises in intra-abdominal pressure. It is also important in emergency situations when the other mechanisms are overwhelmed, as in patients with diarrhoea. Contraction of the external sphincter may prevent soiling in these circumstances.

The puborectalis muscle

The puborectalis muscle (Fig. 12) appears to be of critical importance to the maintenance of faecal continence. Contraction of the puborectalis increases the angulation between the lower rectum and the anus, creating a flap valve effect. The anterior and posterior surfaces of the rectum lie on each other. Any action which increases intra-abdominal pressure will force the anterior wall of the lower rectum against the upper part of the anal canal, thus resisting forward movement of faeces. The anorectal angle is normally 60–105 degrees. Continence is usually lost if the angle exceeds 110 degrees. Continuous activity of the puborectalis, like that of the external sphincter, is mediated by a spinal cord reflex. The puborectalis sling has been considered the most important of the various elements contributing to anal continence but this view has been challenged by those who have been unable to demonstrate the 'flap value' mechanism described above.

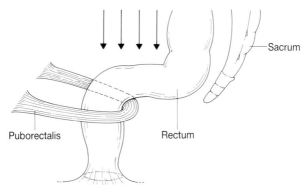

Figure 12 The puborectalis muscle.

The anal cushions

As muscles have a finite length a circular muscle cannot contract sufficiently to close its lumen unless kept under stretch by a thick epithelial and subepithelial internal layer. The anal lining is folded to form highly vascular anal cushions. It has been suggested that at low sphincter pressures these will tend to swell whereas at higher pressures they would be compressed. Thus when the anal canal relaxes this mechanism would contribute to continence by expanding to fill the lumen.

One further mechanism may contribute to the maintenance of faecal continence. Muscular activity is more pronounced in the rectum than in the sigmoid colon. The amplitude of the pressure waves in the rectum is lower than those of the colon but the frequency is greater.

Age-related changes

There are a number of changes in the above mechanisms with increasing age. Rectal motility appears to reduce, as does the strength of contraction of the external sphincter. Reflex contraction of the external sphincter in response to rectal distension is lost in many normal elderly. There is controversy regarding the effect of age on internal sphincter function. Some studies have shown it to reduce with age while others have failed to detect any difference in resting anal pressure with ageing. Anal sensation is also impaired in the elderly. These age-related changes in the mechanisms responsible for the maintenance of faecal continence may contribute to the increased incidence of faecal incontinence in the elderly.

Defecation

Faecal material enters the rectum after a series of colonic mass movements referred to as the gastrocolic reflex. It has been pointed out that this is not gastric or colic or a reflex. It is present in patients who have had a gastrectomy, involves the caecum as well as the colon, and is present even if the nerve supply to the colon is damaged. The main stimuli for these movements appear to be the ingestion of food and physical activity. Small amounts of material in the rectum trigger the accommodation and sampling responses. Larger amounts may trigger the defecation response.

The accommodation response

The entry of sufficient material into the rectum to distend it will cause a rise in the pressure in the rectum, which persists for about a minute. The pressure within the rectum then returns to its previous level. This is known as the accommodation response. With increasing volumes the pressure does not return fully to its pre-inflation level and a gradual increase in rectal pressure occurs. At a variable pressure the urge to defecate is experienced. This passes off as the rectum again accommodates the pressure rise. The accommodation response is usually accompanied by the sampling response.

The sampling response

Rectal distension leads to relaxation of the internal sphincter while at the same time increasing the activity of the external sphincter. This allows the material in the rectum to come into contact with the very sensitive lining of the anus which can discriminate between flatus and liquid or solid faeces. The individual can then choose to resist the passage of any material or to pass flatus or defecate. When rectal distension leads to the urge to defecate, voluntary contraction of the external sphincter, which can be maintained for about a minute, is usually sufficient to allow accommodation to occur in the rectum and thus the urge to defecate is lost. It will not usually return until an additional amount of faeces enters the rectum. This may take a few hours. Should the decision be made to defecate, the defecation response comes into play.

The defecation response

Having decided to accede to the urge to defecate, the individual takes up the squatting position. This has the effect of increasing the anorectal angle. Relaxation of the puborectalis muscle further increases the angle. A Valsalva manoeuvre is performed. The diaphragm moves downward and the abdominal muscles contract with a corresponding rise in intra-abdominal pressure. The internal and external sphincters both relax. Faeces are expelled either as one long unit or as a number of units and expulsion is aided by gravity. Defecation may result in emptying of the rectum or the entire bowel distal to the splenic flexure. Contraction of the rectal muscle is not thought to aid in the expulsion of faeces. The peristaltic wave follows the faecal bolus and is thought to wipe the rectum clean. Defecation is a spinal reflex and is dependent on the integrity of the lumbosacral cord. In patients with higher spinal cord lesions defecation can be triggered reflexly by stimuli such as stroking the perianal region.

Reference

Gibbons CP, Bannister JJ, Trowbridge EA, Read NW. Role of anal cushions in maintaining continence. *Lancet* 1986; **1:** 886–887.

Chapter 10

Faecal incontinence

Faecal incontinence is, fortunately, much less common than urinary incontinence. It affects less than 1 per cent of the elderly within the community. It is much commoner amongst those in institutional care, affecting 10 per cent in residential care and 30 per cent requiring long-term nursing care. Faecal incontinence is particlarly prevalent among confused or immobile patients, the vast majority of whom are also incontinenct of urine. It is understandably less well tolerated by relatives and carers than urinary incontinence. Nursing staff tend to be more upset by the unpredictability of its occurrence than by having to deal with its consequences. It adds significantly to the workload of caring for the patient and they cannot plan for the additional work that will be required. Table 3 lists some of the causes of faecal incontinence in the elderly. Faecal incontinence secondary to diarrhoea, faecal incontinence secondary to faecal impaction and neurological causes of faecal incontinence account for most cases.

Table 3 Causes of faecal incontinence

Diarrhoea
Faecal impaction
Neurological causes
Dementia
Impaired consciousness
Cord lesions
Cauda equina lesions
Idiopathic faecal incontinence
Obstetric trauma
Perineal trauma
Rectal prolapse
Anal surgery
Anal dilatation
Haemorrhoidectomy
Fistula repair
Anal fissure surgery
Drainage of perineal abscesses

Diarrhoea

Any condition causing diarrhoea may lead to faecal incontinence in the elderly. Severe diarrhoea may lead to incontinence at any age but older patients are more likely to suffer from it. It has been suggested that this increased susceptibility is due to neurogenic damage to the anal sphincter mechanism such that anal sphincter function is sufficient to maintain continence under normal conditions but fails when it has to deal with the additional stress of loose stools. Treatment involves identifying and managing the cause of the diarrhoea. Among the conditions that should be considered are infective diarrhoea, neoplastic disease, inflammatory bowel disease, large bowl ischaemia, diverticular disease, thyrotoxicosis and drug therapy (laxatives, antacids).

Faecal impaction

The term faecal impaction is used to indicate the presence of a large mass of hard faeces in the rectum. In some patients the mass is soft rather than hard. Rarely the impacted faeces may be beyond the reach of the examining finger. Faecal impaction complicates constipation in many elderly patients. The rectum of patients with faecal impaction needs to be distended by a much larger volume than normal before the patient senses rectal fullness and has the desire to defecate. These abnormalities allow faeces to accumulate in the rectum. It is believed that elderly patients with faecal impaction are unable to detect the presence of faeces in the rectum until the mass is too large to expel. Confused or depressed patients may ignore the 'call to stool' allowing faeces to accumulate in the rectum. Other factors including immobility and faulty diet may also be important.

Patients with faecal impaction have impaired anal and perianal sensation. They also have a significant increase in the anorectal angle and only in 50 per cent does external sphincter contraction occur in response to rectal distension. Where the response occurs it requires a greater extending volume than normal. In the past the occurrence of faecal incontinence in patients with faecal impaction was thought to be a consequence of stretching of the anal sphincters by the faecal mass or due to reflex inhibition of anal tone by rectal distension. The hard faecal mass was believed to irritate the rectum with resultant increased mucus secretion which then leaked out through the lax sphincters. Both hypotheses have been disproved. There is no significant difference between the sphincter pressures of patients with faecal impaction and age- and sex-matched controls. Nor is there any difference between patients and controls in the rectoanal inhibitory reflex. It has also been shown that basal and maximum squeeze sphincter pressures are unchanged after disimpaction and restoration of continence. It is currently believed that faecal incontinence in patients with faecal impaction is due to the combination of an obtuse anorectal angle, lower anal pressures and impaired anal sensation. As a result of impaired sensation, patients have no warning of impending faecal leakage and are thus unable to prevent it by voluntary contraction of the external sphincter. Whether this impairment of sensation is age-related or secondary to other factors, such as neurological degeneration due to long-term laxative abuse remains to be determined. Loss of anal sensation of itself will not lead to incontinence. Patients in whom the anal canal is anaesthetized using lignocaine gel remain continent. Loss of continence seems to require the co-existence of a number of abnormalities.

Constipation in the elderly has many causes. In any patient it may be multifactorial. Among the causes are immobility, a low-residue diet, dehydration, depression, neoplastic disease, myxoedema, hypercalcaemia, autonomic neuropathy, spinal cord lesions, diverticular disease, partial rectal prolapse and medication (morphine, codeine, anticholinergic agents, antidepressants, antacids, iron).

The management of faecal incontinence due to faecal impaction involves removal of the faecal impaction and prevention of its recurrence. Removal of the impacted faeces usually involves the use of enemas. These have to be given on a daily basis until there is no further response and this may take a week or longer. The mistake made by most nurses is to stop after the first successful enema. Phosphate enemas are usually used for this purpose. These contain sodium acid phosphate which, being poorly absorbed from the bowel, acts osmotically to increase the fluid content of the faeces. The resultant rectal distension induces defecation. If these fail an olive oil enemia may be effective. In some patients the process may have to be initiated by manual evacuation. Where enemas and laxatives fail, more drastic purgatives are available. These include the use of high doses of the osmotic laxative magnesium sulphate, whole gut irrigation with mannitol or polyethylene glycol (Golytely) and a combination of sodium picosulphate and magnesium citrate (Picolax).

Once the impaction has been cleared and continence restored, efforts should be directed towards preventing its recurrence. Where the underlying cause or causes of the impaction can be rectified this should be done but it is not always possible. Immobile, confused elderly patients will re-impact unless appropriate measures are taken. This requires the use of laxatives combined when necessary with regular enemas. Among the laxatives which can be used are the following:

1. Lactulose, a synthetic disaccharide containing one molecule of fructose and one of galactose. It is metabolized in the colon to short-chain organic acids, mainly lactic acid, which alter colonic pH.
2. Docusate sodium (Dioctyl) which lowers the surface tension of faeces, allowing water to penetrate into the faeces.
3. Senna (Senokot), a stimulant laxative which is metabolized by the bacteria in the colon. The metabolite has a direct stimulant effect on the myenteric plexus.
4. Sodium picosulphate (Picolax), a stimulant laxative.
5. Bisacodyl (Dulcolax), a stimulant laxative which stimulates

chemoreceptors in the large bowel with reflex motor effects presumed to involve the myenteric plexus. It can be given orally or as a suppository.

Laxatives alone are ineffective in some patients. Weekly enemas are often the best insurance against further episodes of faecal impaction with its attendant complications. Apart from faecal incontinence, impaction may be complicated by gastrointestinal obstruction, urinary retention, worsening confusion and stercoral ulceration. Stercoral ulcers are due to pressure necrosis of the mucosa of the rectum or colon. They may be asymptomatic but may also lead to rectal haemorrhage or perforation with peritonitis. The last complication may occur during efforts to relieve impaction.

Neurological disease

The central control of defecation is poorly understood. The defecation reflex centres appear to be localized in the sacral cord and cauda equina. Neurological lesions above this level may impair sensation but will not usually impair defecation itself. Urge incontinence of faeces occurs not only in patients with diarrhoea but also in patients with spinal cord and cerebral lesions. Continence of faeces requires that the individual be aware of impending defecation and can inhibit defecation if the time is inconvenient or the place unsuitable. These abilities may be absent in patients with spinal cord lesions or global cerebral disease. In patients with cauda equina lesions sensation is lost and there is no muscle activity whatsoever in the pelvic floor. In patients with suprasacral spinal cord lesions, reflex emptying of the rectum will occur once the stage of spinal shock has passed. Sensation is lost but defecation is usually effective. The patient is incontinent of faeces. Some patients are able to induce defecation by stimulating the lower anal canal.

Many demented patients eventually become incontinent of faeces and in some this will be due to faecal impaction. These patients will tend to be incontintent of frequent small volumes of liquid faeces. Others, however, are not impacted and are incontinent of a large volume of formed faeces once or twice a day. Some of these patients may have lost awareness of the social need to defecate in the appropriate setting. Other possible explanations have been investigated. It has been shown that patients with dementia have multiple uninhibited rectal contractions due to loss of cerebral inhibition. However, it has also been demonstrated that the contribution of these to faecal incontinence in this group of patients is insignificant.

The management of patients with faecal incontinence due to global cerebral disease is based on the principle of induced constipation with periodic planned evacuation. The patient is constipated, for example with codeine phosphate, and then given two or more enemas per week. This regimen ensures that the patient will defecate at predetermined times and is not incontinent in between these. Even where patients are incontinent of faeces after the enema, management is improved because they are only incontinent twice per week, and because the incontinence occurs at a predictable time giving the nursing staff the opportunity to plan for its occurrence. Care must be taken to ensure that the patient has effective enemas otherwise faecal impaction and incontinence will occur. An alternative regimen is to attempt to reinforce the gastrocolic reflex by giving neostigmine (15–30 mg) before meals and then a glycerine suppository about an hour after the meal. If this fails an enema is given.

Idiopathic faecal incontinence

Idiopathic faecal incontinence, also known as anorectal incontinence, is a condition which affects mainly young and middle-aged women. The female to male ratio is 8:1. On examination, patients are found to have a lax sphincter, loss of the anorectal angle and an absent anal reflex. Unlike most elderly patients with faecal incontinence these patients are usually continent of urine. They have evidence of denervation which is most prominent in the external anal sphincter, less prominent in the puborectalis muscle and least prominent in the levator ani muscle. It is believed to result from stretching of the pudendal nerve as a result of a difficult labour or as a result of prolonged excessive straining to defecate. Many female patients give a history of a prolonged second stage of labour or transverse arrest of the fetal head. It has been suggested that the pudendal nerves are damaged by being compressed between the fetal head and the wall of the pelvis. Medical treatment of this condition is to change stool consistency, as patients are less likely to be incontinent when their faeces are firm. Surgical treatment involves recreating the angle between the lower rectum and the upper anal canal. The operation is referred to as post-anal repair. Overall good results are obtained in around 50 per cent of cases.

Other causes of faecal incontinence

Faecal incontinence may also result from obstetric trauma, severe perineal trauma usually sustained in road traffic accidents, and surgical damage to the sphincter. The last may be a complication of anal dilatation, drainage of perineal abscesses, haemorrhoidectomy, fistula repair or fissure surgery. Treatment is surgical, either an external anal sphincter repair or post-anal repair. If these fail other surgical options include anal encirclement with a silver wire, elastic material, skeletal muscle or an artificial implantable anal sphincter.

Repair of a prolapse will restore continence in around two thirds of patients.

Biofeedback has been used with some success in patients with faecal incontinence due to a variety of different causes. They must have some rectal sensation and be able to contract the external anal sphincter voluntarily. It is very labour intensive and requires a well motivated patient. If all else fails the patient quality of life may be improved by a colostomy.

Appropriate history taking and physical examination will identify the cause of faecal incontinence in most cases where needed. Additional information can be obtained by anal manometry, cinedefecography or electromyography.

References

Barrett JA, Brocklehurst JC, Kiff ES, Ferguson G, Farher EB. Anal function in geriatric patients with faecal incontinence. *Gut* 1989; **30:** 1244–1251.

Barrett JA, Brocklehurst JC, Kiff ES, Ferguson G, Faragher EB. Rectal motility studies in faecally incontinent geriatric patients. *Age Ageing* 1990; **19:** 311–318.

Brocklehurst JC, Kirkland JL, Ashford JM. Constipation in long-stay elderly patients: its treatment and prevention by lactulose, poloxalkol-Dihydroxyanthroquinolone and phosphate enemas. *Gerontology* 1983; **29:** 181–184.

Henry MM, Simson JNL. Results of postanal repair: a retrospective study. *Br. J. Surg.* 1985; **72**(suppl.)**:** 17–19.

Keighley MRB, Fielding JWL. Management of faecal incontinence and results of surgical treatment. *Br. J. Surg.* 1983; **70:** 463–468.

Madoff RD, Williams JG, Caushaj PF. Faecal Incontinence. *New England Journal of Medicine* 1992; **326:** 1002–1007.

Parks AG, Swash M, Urich H. Sphincter denervation in anorectal incontinence and rectal prolapse. *Gut* 1977; **18:** 656–665.

Percy JP, Neill ME, Kandiah TK, Swash M. A neurogenic factor in faecal incontinence in the elderly. *Age Ageing* 1982; **11:** 175–179.

Read NW, Abouzekry L. Why do patients with faecal impaction have faecal incontinence. *Gut* 1986; **27:** 283–287.

Read NW, Abouzekry L, Read MG, Howell P, Ottewell D, Donnelly TC. Anorectal function in elderly patients with faecal impaction. *Gastroenterology* 1985; **89:** 959–966.

Tobin GW, Brocklehurst JC. Faecal incontinence in residential homes for the elderly: prevalence, aetiology and management. *Age Ageing* 1986; **15:** 41–46.

Index

Accommodation reflex, 84
Afferent nerves, 4
Age-related changes, 9
  defaecation, 83
  in incidence of incontinence, 26
Alzheimer's disease, 19
  neurogenic bladder in, 22
Anal canal
  anatomy of, 80
  muscles of, 81
Anal cushions, 83
Anal reflex, 82
Anal sensation
  loss of, 88
Anal sphincters, 81
  in defaecation, 84
  nerve supply, 81
  neurological damage, 87
Anal sphincter, external
  age changes in, 83
  in faecal impaction, 87
  repair of, 90
  role in continence, 82
  stimuli, 82
Anal sphincter, internal
  role in continence, 81
Anorectal incontinence, 90
Anterior colporrhaphy, 63
Anticholinergic agents, 53
Augmentation cystoplasty, 66
Autonomic dysreflexia, 23
Autonomous neurogenic bladder, 19

Behaviour therapy, 48
Bethanechol chloride, 60
Biofeedback in treatment, 49
Bladder
  anatomy of, 1–2

calculi, 16, 43, 76
distension, 68
filling rate, 7, 36
low-compliance, 12
motor paralytic, 20
neoplasms of, 16
nerves of, 3
neuropathic
  See neurogenic bladder
overdistension of, 14, 17
pressure measurement, 35, 36
pressure-volume relationships, 36
sympathetic nerve supply, 20
Bladder capacity, 37
  effect of age, 9
  measurement of, 37
Bladder compliance, 37
Bladder contractions, 6
  involuntary, 12
Bladder drill, 48–9, 57
  in males, 49
Bladder instability
  surgery for, 62, 64
  See also Detrusor instability
Bladder neck
  action of, 6
  opening mechanism, 8
  repositioning of, 62
  in stress incontinence, 16
Bladder neck dyssynergia, 43
Bladder neck suspensions, 63
Bladder tone, 7
Bladder transection, 67
Bladder washouts for encrustation, 75
Bromocriptine, 57
Burch colposuspension, 63

Calcium antagonists, 53

Carbachol, 60
Catheters and catheterization, 72–7
  bypassing of urine, 72, 76
  classification of, 73
  complications, 74
  encrustation in, 75
  infection from, 73, 74
  intermittent self-, 23, 76
  rejection of, 76
  suprapubic, 76
Cauda equina lesions
  defaecation and, 89
Cerebral disease
  faecal incontinence in, 89
Cerebrovascular disease, 19, 79
  causing neurogenic bladder, 21
Cervical radiculopathy, 19
Cholinergic agents, 60
Clam cystoplasty, 66
Collecting devices, 73
Constipation, 87
  causes, 88
  laxatives for, 88
Cystitis, interstitial, 12, 16
Cystocele, 63
Cystomat, 68
Cystometry, 36, 42
Cystoscopy, 40

Defaecation
  accommodation reflex, 84
  age changes, 8
  central control of, 89
  mechanism of, 83
  physiology of, 80–5
  sampling response, 84
  in spinal cord lesions, 85
Defaecation reflex, 89
Defaecation response, 84
Dementia, 66
  faecal incontinence in, 89
  prompted voiding in, 48
Depression, 27, 88
Detrusor 1
  coordination with urethra, 5
  reflex inhibition of, 72
  tone, 7
  transection of, 67
Detrusor areflexia, 17, 20
Detrusor contraction
  agents affecting, 60, 61
  impaired, 14, 30
  prostaglandins affecting, 60
  prostaglandin inhibitors affecting, 57

Detrusor hyperreflexia, 12, 13, 14
  bladder distension in 68
  cerebral cortical lesions causing, 20
  cystoplasty for, 66
  in diabetes, 21
  drug therapy, 53
  management of, 46
  in multiple sclerosis, 21
  sacral neurectomy for, 67
  in spinal cord trauma, 22
  voiding regime for, 50
Detrusor instability, 13, 14, 21
  as psychosomatic problem, 27, 50
  biofeedback in, 49
  bladder distension for, 68
  bladder drill in, 48, 49, 50
  cystoplasty for, 66
  diagnosis, 31
  drug therapy, 53
  idiopathic, 48, 49, 50
  management of, 46
  mechanism of, 13
  pad tests in, 33
  pressure studies, 37, 38
  psychological aspects of, 27
  surgery for, 62, 63, 65
  urodynamic studies in, 41, 42, 43, 44
  with neurological lesion, 44
  with outflow obstruction, 65
Detrusor sphincter dyssnergia, 5, 18, 20
  cerebral lesions causing, 20, 21
  in multiple sclerosis, 21
  in spinal cord lesions, 22
  surgery of, 68
Detrusor under-activity, 14, 17, 58, 60
  diagnosis of, 35
Diabetes mellitus, 20
  causing neurogenic bladder, 20, 21
  unstable detrusor in, 12
Diagnosis of incontinence, 28–45, 52
  accuracy of, 31
  problems of, 30
Diarrhoea, 86–7
Distigmine bromide, 60
Drug treatment, 52–61
  agents for, 58
  efficacy of, 52
  side-effects of, 53, 55, 60

Efferent parasympathetic nerve supply, 3
Efferent pathways, 5
Efferent somatic nerve supply, 4
Efferent sympathetic nerve supply, 3
Electrical therapy, 71

Electromyography, 39
Emepromium bromide, 56
Encrustation of catheters, 75
Enemas for faecal impaction, 88
Environment, 79
Ephedrine in stress incontinence, 59
Epidemiology, 25–6
Epididymo-orchitis, 76
Established incontinence, 11

Faecal continence, 89
    maintenance of, 81
Faecal impaction, 18, 87–9
    causing incontinence, 11, 87
    management of, 88
Faecal incontinence, 86–91
    causes of, 86
    in faecal impaction, 11, 87
    idiopathic, 90
    incidence of, 86
    management of, 88, 89
    obstetric trauma causing, 90
Faecal urge incontinence, 89
Faradism, 71
Fistulae, 17, 73
Flavoxate, 56
Frequency of micturition, 12, 16, 18, 49
    definition of, 12
    diagnosis of, 30
    in outflow tract obstruction, 43
    with stress incontinence, 31
Frequency volume charts, 32
Functional incontinence, 17

Garments, protective, 77
Gastrocolic reflex, 84, 90
Gastrointestinal tract
    anatomy of, 80
Geriatric wards
    incidence of incontinence in, 26
    timed voiding in, 46

Habit retraining, 47
Handwashing incontinence, 14
Histamine, 61
5-Hydroxytrypramine, 61
Hypnotherapy, 50

Imipramine, 49, 56
Incidence of urinary incontinence, 25
Incontinence, faecal
    See Faecal incontinence

Incontinence, urinary
    See also types etc
    causes, 10
    definitions, 10, 25
    mechanism of, 6
    pathophysiology of, 10–24
Inflammatory bowel disease, 87
Interstitial cystitis, 12, 16
Intrautethral pressure, 4
Intravenous urogram, 35
Involuntary urethral relaxation, 12

Kanga pants, 78

Large bowel ischaemia, 87
Laxatives, 87, 88
Long routing detrusor reflex, 5, 6
Low-compliance bladder, 12

Marshall-Marchetti-Kranz operation, 63
Micturition
    See also Voiding
    control of, 5, 6
    physiology of, 6–9
    spinal cord and, 5
Micturition reflex, 7
Molyncke pants, 78
Motor paralytic bladder, 20
Motor urgency, 13
Mucosal seal mechanism, 8, 59
Multiple sclerosis, 19
    neurogenic bladder in, 21
Myxoedema, 88

Neostigmine reinforcing gastrocolic
    reflex, 90
Nerve supply to urinary tract, 3
Nerve varicosities, 4
Neurogenic bladder, 12, 18–23
    autonomous, 19
    diseases causing, 20
    reflex, 19
    sensory, 19
    uninhibited, 19
    with detrusor instability, 44
    with outflow tract obstruction, 65
Nocturia, 12, 49
    diagnosis of, 30
    in outflow tract obstruction, 43
    with stress incontinence, 31
Norfenefrine, 59

Obstetric trauma causing faecal
    incontinence, 90

Oestrogens in stress incontinence, 59
Outflow obstruction, 13, 18, 30
  detrusor instability and, 65
  diagnosis, 43
  neurological lesion with, 65
  operative intervention for, 44, 65
  prostatic, 35
  stents for, 65

Ovarian cysts, 18
Oxybutynin hydrochloride, 56, 76
  side effects of, 54
  treatment with, 54

Pad tests, 33
Parkinson's disease, 19, 21, 65, 79
Pathophysiology of incontinence, 10–24
Pelvic floor muscles, 4, 72
  electrical stimulation of, 77
  exercises, 70
Penile gangrene, 73
Pereyra operation, 64
Perinometer, 71
Perinicious anaemia, 20
Phenol
  trigonal injection of, 67
Phenylpropanolamine, 59
Physiotherapy, 70–2
Post-menopausal atrophy
  causing stress incontinence, 15
Post-prostatectomy incontinence, 16, 59
  physiotherapy in, 70
Post-prostatectomy stress incontinence,
    59
  Teflon injections for, 64
Pressure flow studies, 38
Pressure measurements, 35–8
  urethral, 36
Prompted voiding, 48
Propantheline, 56
Prostaglandins, 60
Prostaglandin inhibitors, 53, 57–8
Prostate
  carcinoma of, 18
  size of, 30
  transurethral resection, 16
Prostatectomy
  incontinence following
    See Post-prostatectomy incontinence
Prostatic hypertrophy, 13, 18, 24, 43
Protective garments, 77
Psychological aspects, 26–8
Puborectalis muscle
  in faecal incontinence, 82

Radiotherapy
  causing incontinence, 12
  sensory urgency following, 16
Rectal carcinoma, 20
Rectal examination, 29, 30
Rectal prolapse, 88
Rectum
  anatomy of, 80
  in continence, 81
  distension, 81
  pressure measurements, 35
Reflex incontinence, 12
Reflex neurogenic bladder, 19
Residential care
  incidence of incontinence in, 26
  incidence of faecal incontinence in, 86
  staff attitudes, 27
  timed voiding in, 46
Retropubic surgery, 63
Rhabdosphincter, 3, 36

Sacral neurectomy, 66
Sampling response, 84
Senile dementia, 22
  See also Alzheimer's disease
Sensory neurogenic bladder, 19
Sensory urge incontinence, 11
Sensory urgency, 16
Sex differences in incontinence, 26
Sexual difficulties, 27
Smooth muscle relaxants, 53
Sphincters
  artificial, 64
Sphincter bradykinesia, 21
Sphincter mechanism, 9
  in stress incontinence, 15
  repair of, 62
Spinal cord
  micturition control and, 5
  tumours of, 19
  lesions, 22, 85, 89
Stamey operation, 64
Stents for outflow obstruction, 65
Stress incontinence, 13, 14
  artificial sphincters for, 64
  biofeedback for, 50
  bladder neck in, 16
  combined transvaginal and retropubic
    procedures, 64
  definition of, 14
  diagnosis of, 30, 31, 32
  drug therapy, 58, 59–60
  in male, 16, 43, 59, 64
  pad tests in, 33

Stress incontinence – *cont.*
  physiotherapy in, 71
  post-prostatectomy, 59, 64
  pressure studies, 36, 38
  retropubic surgery for, 63
  sling operations for, 64
  sphincter mechanism in, 15
  surgery for, 62–4
  Teflon injections for, 64
  types of, 15
  types of surgery for, 63
  urodynamic studies in, 40, 41, 42
  vaginal approach to surgery, 63
  VCU in, 39
Strokes, 21
Struvite in catheters, 75
Subtrigonal phenol injection, 67
Suprapubic catheterization, 76
Surgical treatment, 62–9
Sympathetic nerve supply, 4

Tabes dorsalis, 20, 82
Teflon injections for stress incontinence,
  64
Terodiline, 55
Thyrotoxicosis, 87
Timed voiding, 46–7
Toileting behaviour
  individual, 46
  modification of, 48
Transient urinary incontinence, 10
Transverse myelitis, 19
Trigone, 1, 59
Tuberculous cystitis, 12

Ultrasound in diagnosis, 40
Ureteric orifices, 1
Ureters during voiding, 7
Urethra
  anatomy of, 2
  as sphincter, 6
  coordination with detrusor, 5
  dilatation of, 2
  diverticulae, 73
  electromyography, 39
  failure of support, 15
  female, 2, 3
  function, 8–9
  involuntary relaxation, 12
  male, 2, 3
  mucosal seal mechanism, 8
  nerve supply, 3
  pressure, 4, 8
  pressure measurements, 35

  resting pressure, 8
  stricture, 76
  surgical compression, 63
  unstable, 14, 16
Urethral closure pressure, 8, 9
Urethral pressure profile, 36
Urethral resistance, 62
Urethritis
  atrophic, 59
Urge incontinence, 12, 13, 65
  bladder drill in, 49
  diagnosis, 30, 32
  urodynamic studies, 40
  with stress incontinence, 31
Urge incontinence of faeces, 89
Urgency, 16, 18, 30
  in outflow tract obstruction, 43
Urinary flow rates, 33
  age changes, 9
  female, 35
  male, 35
  measurement of, 33, 34
Urinary incontinence
  See Incontinence
Urinary retention, 60
Urinary tract
  age-related changes in, 9
  anatomy and physiology, 1
  peripheral innervation, 3–6
Urinary tract function
  filling phase, 6
  micturition
    See Micturition
  neural control of, 4
  phases of, 6
Urinary tract infections
  catheters causing, 73, 74
  causing incontinence, 11
  cystometry causing, 42
  sensory urgency in, 16
Urine
  bypassing, 72, 76
  collecting bags, 73
  nocturnal excretion, 9
  sensory urgency in, 16
  residual, 32, 33
Urodynamic investigations, 29, 32–45
  ambulatory, 39
  definition of, 32
  on elderly patients, 23
  indications in female, 40
  indications in male, 43
Uterus
  fibroids in, 18

Vaginal examination, 29
Vaginal surgery for stress incontinence, 63
Vasoactive intestinal polypeptide, 4, 14, 61
Vesicovaginal fistula, 17
Videocystourethrography (VCU), 38–9
Voiding
   See also Micturition
   age changes in, 9
   bladder function during, 7
   deferment of, 7
   initiation of, 8
   prompted, 48
   timed, 46
   ureters during, 7
Voiding disorder, 17
   diagnosis of, 30, 31
   in female, 17
Voiding regimes, 46–51
   individual, 47
   timed, 46